BIO-IDENTICAL HORMONES AND TELOMERASE

BIO-IDENTICAL HORMONES AND TELOMERASE

The Nobel Prize–Winning Research into Human Life Extension and Health

Dr. Edmund Chein, M.D., J.D., and
Dr. Hiroshi Demura, M.D., Ph.D.

iUniverse, Inc.
Bloomington

Bio-identical Hormones and Telomerase
The Nobel Prize–Winning Research into Human Life Extension and Health

iUniverse books may be ordered through booksellers or by contacting:

iUniverse
1663 Liberty Drive
Bloomington, IN 47403
www.iuniverse.com
1-800-Authors (1-800-288-4677)

ISBN: 978-1-4502-5577-6 (sc)
ISBN: 978-1-4502-5575-2 (hc)
ISBN: 978-1-4502-5576-9 (e)

Printed in the United States of America
iUniverse rev. date: 09/20/2011

CONTENTS

PREFACE

In 2009, the Nobel Committee awarded the Nobel Prize in Medicine to three scientists in the field of telomere and telomerase research.

Telomeres are present in every cell in the body. They comprise the tail portion of our DNA, which controls the cell's lifespan. These three scientists proved that when the telomeres are long, the cell is young and can replicate into youthful daughter cells. When the telomeres are short, the cell replicates into old, ugly cells and gradually dies. The scientists showed how telomerase works to lengthen the telomere portion of our DNA and thus achieve youthful cell replications and perpetual non-dying cells in the laboratory.

The telomeres in our DNA are controlled by the telomerase enzyme. The telomerase, in turn, is controlled by the hormones in our body.

This knowledge is important to our health because we can now *foretell* the onset of an age-related disease *before* it happens by looking at the length of the telomeres in the cells. For example, we can foretell the onset of cancer by looking at the telomeres of lymphocytes, and we can spot an impending heart attack by looking at the telomeres of the heart muscle. Since telomeres are controlled by telomerase, and telomerase is controlled by our hormones, we can also foretell and *prevent* the onset of age-related diseases by checking our hormones regularly. Keeping the telomeres in our DNA long by optimizing our hormones can *stop the ravages of disease* in our bodies and will *enable us to stay young.*

Hormones are body secretions that function like e-mails, faxes, or letters from one organ to another, telling the other organs what to do. There are two types of hormones. One type is *bio-identical*, so called because they are identical to the ones made in our bodies. The other type of hormone is *synthetic*, which are actually drugs or chemicals that scientists and doctors use to treat diseases. A blood test can be used to check one's bio-identical hormones, and this can be done by any laboratory with a doctor's order. The synthetic chemical hormones are the ones that cause cancer and are *not* checked by any laboratories.

Did you know that your body is the Temple of the Holy Spirit? It is, according to 1 Corinthians 6:20. My question to you is, when did you last have your hormone levels checked for your Temple?

If you recount how much money you spent last year on making yourself look good, on your house, on your cars, then compare that to the amount you spent on checking the condition of your Temple, you might be ashamed. When we get seriously sick, we ask God, "Why does this happen to me?" But God might say to you, "Do you check your Temple as often as you check your car?" When it comes to having their Temples checked, many people are in the habit of saying, "Is that paid by my health insurance? If it is I will do the test, but if it is *not*, I will not." Do you say that when you have your car checked?

Palm Springs Life Extension Institute, founded by Dr. Chein in 1994, was the first clinic in the United States to offer human growth hormone to lengthen the telomeres in the cells of normal adults. Now there are more than 4,000 doctors in the United States doing this procedure.

In 2005, proof was obtained that growth hormone acts directly on the telomerase, which in turn lengthens the telomere of the DNA (see Dr. Sanchez's work below). Today we also have the validation of the Nobel Committee that keeping our telomeres long is important in preventing the cells from getting old or diseased, and it is the scientific way of achieving longevity.

TELOMERASE ACTIVATING THERAPY: A FIELD THAT RECEIVED THE 2009 NOBEL PRIZE IN MEDICINE

The details of Telomerase Activating Therapy were originally described in my book *Age Reversal*, first published in January 1998. There I described the mechanism in which bio-identical hormones play a role in activating telomerase, which in turn prolongs the telomere portion of our DNA. This process keeps the cell young and healthy, thus accomplishing our goal of staying healthy, young, and achieving longevity. In 2009, the Nobel Committee validated this process by awarding the Nobel Prize in Medicine to three scientists who showed how telomerase works to lengthen the telomere portion of our DNA and thus achieves youthful cell replications and perpetual non-dying cells in the laboratory.

Even though the prize went to three scientists, thousands more deserve to share the prize, especially the group at the University of Texas, Southwest Division, who reached the amazing goal of making human cells live "forever" in laboratory conditions (*Science*, Vol. 279, January 16, 1998).

My respect also goes to the following scientists:

- Dr. Gomez Sanchez and his group at La Paz University, Spain, who showed that growth hormone directly activates telomerase (*Journal of Endocrinology*, Vol. 185, June 2005, pages 421–428). This is exactly why growth hormone has become popularly used to lengthen the telomeres of DNA.
- Dr. Scott Brouilette and his group, who showed that telomere length is a predictor of the onset of coronary heart disease (*Lancet*, Vol. 369, January 13, 2007).
- Dr. Xu and his group at the National Institutes of Health and the University of Utah, who showed that the use of multivitamins is associated with longer telomere length among women (*AM Journal of Clinical Nutrition*, Vol. 89, 2009, pages 1857–1863). Yes, they validated our practice over the last fifteen years of prescribing daily multivitamins and multiminerals to our patients.
- Drs. Williams and Boggess at the University of North Carolina, who showed that progesterone (not progestin or Medroxy-progesterone) inhibits endometrial telomerase activity, validating the position for years that progesterone inhibits and prevents breast, uterine, and prostate cancers (*Journal of Clinical Endocrinology and Metabolism*, Vol. 86, August 2001, pages 3912–3917).
- Dr. Kaszubowska at the University of Gdansk, Poland, who showed that centenarians have long telomeres in

their cells (lymphocytes). This proves the position that lengthening telomeres *does not* cause cancer (*Journal of Physiology and Pharmacology*, December 2008, Vol. 9, pages 169–186).

- The scientists at the Johns Hopkins University School of medicine who first showed that the bio-identical male hormone testosterone activates telomerase and lengthens telomeres.
- Last but not least, Dr. Michael Sheppard, Vice-Dean of the University of Birmingham Medical School, who says: "Growth hormone therapy *does not* induce cancer" (*Endocrinology and Metabolism*, October 2005, Vol. 2, No. 10, page 57).

For more understanding of the actions of various hormones that activate telomerase, go to the following chapters.

CHAPTER 1

The Youth Quest: From Hormones to Telomeres

RUNNING FASTER, GOING SLOWER

As we grow older, many of us experience a tremendous amount of frustration because something inside us doesn't work the way it used to. Nutrition experts tell us to eat certain kinds of food. Other health experts tell us to get more sleep. Some claim free radicals are the sole cause of aging, and that the only way to longevity is through antioxidant supplements. Fitness gurus tell us the only answer is exercise. When we do exercise or go on a diet, we feel a little better—but not much, and not the way we felt when we were younger. We exercise or diet twice as much to stay at the same place, and even that is a challenge.

The story has been the same throughout history, so we wonder if we should continue to fight the battle, or if we should just learn to grow old gracefully.

THE QUEST FOR YOUTH

Long life—and more importantly, long youth—has been sought after for thousands of years. From ancient times to the present, humans have been searching for a way to live forever—to be immortal. Some cultures believed immortality was contained in an elixir of the gods. Chinese myths tell of a peach from the gods that, if eaten, would grant eternal life. Alexander the Great purportedly went to India to search for the legendary River of Immortal Life. Most of us are familiar with Ponce de León, the Spanish explorer who searched for the Fountain of Youth, a magical spring that would restore youth and health to all who bathed in it.

In our more modern world, we have stopped looking for fountains on mysterious islands. Now we look to medicine to help us live longer. In 1796, Edward Jenner tested his theory that the cowpox virus could provide immunity to the smallpox virus, and the first vaccine was born. One hundred fifty years later, the work of Albert Sabin and Jonas Salk led to vaccines for polio. Since that time, many other killer diseases have been tamed using the same method, so the vaccine can be considered one of the most potent magic elixirs of the early twentieth century.

CHANGING LIFE SPANS

From vaccines to genetic engineering, technology continues to progress and develop at lightning speed. Our knowledge is increasing at such an exponential rate that the idea of living one hundred twenty, one hundred fifty, or one hundred seventy-five years is not science fiction anymore. In another generation, lifespans like these could be everyday reality!

Medical technology is helping to prolong life with developments in antibiotics, microscopic techniques, laser surgery, and organ replacements. What we have learned has helped greatly in our search for youth and long life. The proof lies in the fact that people now live longer. In 1900, the life expectancy for an average person was forty-seven years. By 1985, that life expectancy had risen to almost seventy-five years. Today, the number is closer to seventy-eight years. Not only has life expectancy increased, but the quality of life has improved as well. Today, nearly 80 percent of people sixty-five and older report no disabilities, and these numbers continue to rise dramatically. Today, many people stay mentally and physically sound well into their old age.

Improvements in medical technology and new knowledge about exercise, nutrition, and rest are all part of the solution to remaining young and healthy. However, we continue to see some people who do not take particularly good care of themselves, yet are aging more gently—and we know instinctively that parts of the antiaging puzzle must still be missing.

TELOMERES: THE MISSING PUZZLE PIECE

One missing piece in the antiaging puzzle is an astonishing part of our chromosomes called the *telomere.* New antiaging research shows that aging can now actually be reversed at the cellular level by changing this newly discovered part of our chromosomes. If you aren't yet familiar with the word telomere, you have been missing some of the most revolutionary antiaging research to have come along in years.

Telomeres are structures on the ends of the forty-six chromosomes found inside the human cell. These structures are different in substance and appearance from the rest of the chromosome and have been described as looking like the plastic tips on the ends of shoelaces. Like the tips on shoelaces, they protect the larger structure from damage.

Unlike the tip of a shoelace, however, telomeres protect the chromosome by sacrificing a portion of themselves each time the cell divides. In younger cells, an enzyme called *telomerase,* produced by the telomerase gene, keeps resetting the aging clock by encouraging the telomeres to rebuild themselves, thereby protecting the cell. But as we age, telomerase enzyme levels decrease, and the telomeres shorten with each cell division instead. Eventually, the telomeres become so short that the cells stop dividing and become functionally dead, or senescent. Cell senescence is a significant factor in age-related conditions and diseases.

Researchers have now found that if telomerase genes can once again be prodded to make telomerase, then the telomeres, chromosome, and cell can all be given a new lease on life.[1] To do this, a cell has to go beyond its Hayflick limit. A cell's Hayflick limit is the number of times it will divide before dying. If a cell's Hayflick limit is fifty, for example, it will divide fifty times and then wither and die. When enough of the cells in an organ die, the organ begins to die, too, often with drastic health consequences for the organ's owner.

Scientists have now shown that with the enzyme telomerase present, cells can defy their Hayflick limit and stay alive forever. In lab experiments reported in January 1998, human cells that had been prompted to make telomerase had elongated telomeres, continued to divide vigorously, and exceeded their normal lifespan by at least twenty doublings. These revitalized cells then displayed all the characteristics of young, healthy cells, including an absence of cancer. This was in contrast to normal cells, which exhibited

---

1 Bryan TM, Reddel RR. "Telomere dynamics and telomerase activity in in vitro immortalised human cells." *Eur J Cancer* 33(5):767–773, 1997.

normal telomere shortening, a normal Hayflick limit, and normal cell senescence, or death.[2]

Such research not only suggests that telomeres are the biological clock for cellular aging, but also shows that the clock can be reset. The lifespan of such cells, including their reproductive capabilities, can, under such circumstances, go on forever, and give us our first clear understanding of the cellular mechanism of aging.[3] We may soon be able to determine if these processes can be halted or reversed while at work inside a human being. This scientific breakthrough has unprecedented and profound implications for all aspects of longevity and antiaging medicine.

It stands to reason that if telomeres shorten too early and allow the cell to be damaged, disease or disability of some kind will follow. Several researchers recently pursued this avenue of logic and looked for consistently shortened telomeres in specific diseases. Shortened telomeres were found in many age-related and degenerative diseases, and many non age-related diseases, such as aplastic anemia, ataxia telangiectasia, ulcerative colitis, and Hodgkin's disease.[4]

---

2 Bodnar AG, Ouellette M, Frolkis M, et al. "Extension of life-span by introduction of telomerase into normal human cells." *Science* 279(5349):349–352, 1998.

3 Fossel M. "Telomerase and the aging cell: implications for human health." *JAMA* 279(21):1732–1735, Jun 1998.

4 Metcalfe JA, Parkhill J, Campbell L, et al. "Accelerated telomere shortening in ataxia telangiectasia." *Nat Genet* 13(3):350–353, 1996.

Kinouchi Y, Hiwatashi N, Chida M, et al. "Telomere shortening in the colonic mucosa of patients with ulcerative colitis." *J Gastroenterol* 33(3):343–348, 1998.

Norrback KF, Enblad G, Erlanson M, et al. "Telomerase Activity in Hodgkin's Disease." *Blood* 92(2):567–573, 1998.

Ball SE, Gibson FM, Rizzo S, et al. "Progressive telomere shortening in aplastic anemia." *Blood* 91(10):3582–3592, 1998.

As a result of telomere research, aging is now known to begin earlier in life than formerly believed. These findings were illustrated by an ABC *20/20* investigative news report about telomeres. On January 16, 1998, *20/20* anchor Hugh Downs and his twenty-seven-year-old grandson had their telomeres tested. Not surprisingly, 70 percent of seventy-six-year-old Downs's telomeres were gone. What was surprising was that Downs's twenty-seven-year-old grandson had already lost 40 percent of his.

WHAT ARE TELOMERES AND TELOMERASE?

Every cell in our bodies has a nucleus, and every nucleus has a strand of DNA, the genetic information from our parents. The DNA strand has a tail, and this tail region is called a telomere.

The telomere is like the tip of a shoelace. The function of the tip is to protect the shoelace.

It has been discovered that when the telomere is long, the cell is healthy. When the healthy cell replicates, it replicates into healthy daughter cells. When the telomere is short, the cell ages. Aging of the cell causes disease. When the aged cell replicates, it gives birth to ugly, sick daughter cells. When the telomere disappears, the cell dies.

The discovery that was awarded the 2009 Nobel Prize in Medicine showed us that we now have the scientific ability to lengthen the telomere. We also now have the ability to keep *any* human cell *perpetually alive*. In other words, we have found "the fountain of youth."

Scientists have also found that telomerase itself is controlled and activated by bio-identical hormones (as differentiated from designer hormones). Therefore, in order to keep ourselves healthy and have quality of life, we must maintain all our age-declining bio-identical hormones at optimal levels. Letting those hormones drop is to let the telomeres get short. When the telomeres get short, the cells age. Aging causes disease, and death follows.

If we keep our telomeres long, our cells and bodies remain healthy. When the cells replicate, they give rise to healthy, young daughter cells, and we successfully avoid age-related diseases. Longevity naturally and logically follows.

One example that demonstrates the work of telomerase is to compare the skin cells of a ninety-year-old woman with those of a ten-year-old child. The facial cells of both have a life span of approximately ninety days, after which they are shed and replaced by new skin cells. Question: If the cells on both of their faces have the same life span, why do those of the ninety-year-old looked so wrinkled, and those of the ten-year-old look so beautiful and healthy?

The answer is the work of the telomere. In the ninety-year-old, the telomeres in the skin cells are short, so they give birth to diseased new daughter cells and wrinkled skin. In the ten-year-old, the telomeres in the cells are long, so the cells give birth to healthy daughter cells and beautiful skin.

TELOMERASE ACTIVATING THERAPY

Now that we know how early the aging process starts, how can we use this astounding research to preserve our life-protecting telomeres, when telomerase therapy may not become commercially available for another ten years? Well, even before scientists discovered the effects of telomerase on telomeres, they already knew hormones were a piece of the antiaging puzzle. During the research on telomeres, they may have found out why: certain hormones appear to impact the activity of the telomerase gene.

It appears that the telomerase gene has hormone receptors. It is our belief that all hormones have receptors on the telomerase, which tell the gene whether to continue repairing the cell. Therefore, when the hormone molecules are adequate in number, the telomerase molecule gets the message that the person is young, and it continues to repair the telomere portion of the DNA. When the hormone molecules are low in number, however, the telomerase protein molecule gets the message that the host is old, and it slows down or stops the repair of the telomere portion of the DNA, which causes the cell to become aged.

Various studies have shown that hormone-dependent regulation of telomerase is a reality. One study at Johns Hopkins using testosterone hormones to regulate telomerase activity in the stem cells of the rat prostate represents the first proof for the hormonal regulation of telomerase activity.[5] Several other studies done on human endometrial cells showed that the telomerase activity of the endometrium may be regulated by estrogen hormones. In benign endometrial tissue from premenopausal women, 100 percent showed strong telomerase activity, whereas in post-menopausal women, 100 percent showed weak telomerase activity. Researchers concluded that "the hormone-dependent regulation of telomerase suggests the possibility of therapeutic strategies through hormones that regulate telomerase activity."[6]

---

5 Meeker AK, Sommerfeld HJ, Coffey DS. "Telomerase is activated in the prostate and seminal vesicles of the castrated rat." *Endocrinology* 137(12):5743–5746, 1996.

6 Saito T, Schneider A, Martel N, et al. "Proliferation-associated regulation of telomerase activity in human endometrium and its potential implication in early cancer diagnosis." *Biochem Biophys Res Commun* 231(3):610–614, 1997.

Brien TP, Kallakury BV, Lowry CV, et al. "Telomerase activity in benign endometrium and endometrial carcinoma." *Cancer Res* 57(13):2760–2764, 1997.

Yokoyama Y, Takahashi Y, Morishita S, et al. "Telomerase activity in the human endometrium throughout the menstrual cycle." *Mol Hum Reprod* 4(2):173–177, 1998.

In other studies tracking telomerase production across the course of women's menstrual cycles, higher levels of telomerase were exhibited in the phases corresponding to higher hormone production. Lower levels of telomerase were exhibited in phases of the menstrual cycle associated with lower hormone production. This led the researchers to conclude, "Telomerase is a regulated enzyme linked to cellular proliferation, and hormone functions may be involved in its regulation."[7]

Hormones other than the sex hormones have also been implicated in the regulation of telomerase. In studies done at the University of California, Davis, certain strains of cultured human epidermal (skin) cells were being tested for their reactions to various substances. One of these substances was a hormone called the epidermal growth factor. The epidermal growth factor dramatically stimulated telomerase activity, adding more weight to the growing belief that hormones are the only substances we currently have available to us that can help us keep our telomeres long, young, and healthy.[8]

While science is in the earliest stages of discovery about our telomeres and telomerase, the growing body of evidence shows a definite link between hormones and telomerase. Hormones are not only the first substances scientists looked at, they are also the only ones currently available to us for regulating this antiaging enzyme.

---

7 Kyo S, Takakura M, Kohama T, Inoue M. "Telomerase activity in human endometrium." *Cancer Res* 57(4):610–614, 1997.

8 Rea MA, Phillips MA, Degraffenried LA, et al. "Modulation of human epidermal cell response to 2,3,7,8-tetrachlorodibenzo-p-dioxin by epidermal growth factor." *Carcinogenesis* 19(3):479–483, 1998.

WHAT ARE BIO-IDENTICAL HORMONES?

Hormones are protein molecules secreted by cells in our bodies. They carry a message telling another cell or another organ what to do, like a letter, fax, or e-mail.

Hormones are generally divided into two types:

1. Bio-identical hormones, which are identical to the ones in our bodies. They are identical in terms of chemical structure and biological functions. These hormones are safe to supplement when their levels are low, as long as there is no overdose. (Even an overdose of food or water can cause harm, let alone hormones.)
2. "Designer" hormones, so called because they do not exist in nature. They are designed and created by a scientist or pharmaceutical company. These drugs act like hormones. They almost always cause harm or cancer when taken long-term (with the exception, perhaps, of birth control pills).

Almost all hormones require a prescription by a doctor under federal law in the US. The only exceptions are DHEA, melatonin, pregnenolone, and thymus proteins.

However, *only* bio-identical hormones can activate telomerase. Designer drug-like hormones cannot communicate at all with telomerase. Therefore, they have no place in maintaining youth or creating longevity.

One easy way to tell if the hormone you are taking is bio-identical is to take the name off the label of your bottle and ask a hospital or medical laboratory to test the level of this substance in your body. If the hospital or laboratory can perform the test, the hormone you are taking is bio-identical, because hospitals and laboratories commonly perform tests on hormones in our bodies for our doctors. If the hospital or laboratory cannot or will not perform the test, it must be a designer drug, because doctors normally do not test the level of designer drugs in our bodies.

It is very important to periodically check the levels of bio-identical hormones that control aging. It should be part of our annual physical check-up, like cholesterol and blood sugar. A disease may manifest in the form of high or low hormone levels many years before the disease becomes clinically apparent.

Keeping our bio-identical hormones optimal will keep our telomeres long, and long telomeres keep us healthy and young.

AGING AS A DISORDER

The link between the decline in hormone levels and physical dysfunction has opened the door to a new way of thinking and, most importantly, a new way of looking at aging. We can see now that hormone imbalance is not a result of aging—aging is a result of imbalanced hormones. Couple this with our telomeres shortening themselves into nonexistence, and we have a disorder that begs to be treated.

By accepting the view that aging is a disorder, we open the door to accepting treatment and eventually finding a cure. As with most other disorders, if not treated, aging leads to death. Who wouldn't advise someone who had been diagnosed with cancer to seek treatment? But until the research and medical discoveries of the last two or three years, it sounded crazy to most people to go to a doctor to find a cure for your old age. After all, isn't aging, accompanied by all of its weakness, fatigue, and illness, just an inevitable part of life?

It doesn't have to be. As with diabetes, menopause, and hypothyroidism, the cure for aging lies in balancing the hormones in the body. We have proven that you don't have to lie down and die gracefully because your birth certificate says you are old. You can fight aging and live a long, healthy life filled with the activities you love. With the knowledge we have, it doesn't make sense to give in to fatigue and the other effects of aging. We no longer have to retire to a sedentary life, and then wait to die.

In recent years, research has led to a generally accepted practice of replacing hormones to fight aging and the symptoms that go along with it. We can list the amazing benefits that these hormones provide for the body if replaced in the right amount, but the real proof comes from the thousands of users who report increased energy, less illness, a better sex life, and an overall rejuvenation and newfound excitement for life.

If we want to preserve our telomeres and keep our bodies healthy and youthful, perhaps it makes sense to first take a closer look at the natural, youth-giving magic of hormones.

CHAPTER 2

The Natural Magic of Hormones

The Palm Springs Life Extension Institute was founded in 1994, but I and my associates at the Institute have been engaged in hormone research, both in Japan and in the United States, for more than twenty years. We are becoming more and more convinced that hormone research is leading us into new territory regarding the core of human life itself. The research on hormones has been focused on establishing causes and producing cures for human illnesses, but gradually the focus has shifted to the fundamental improvement of human vitality.

Because hormones make up the source of human vitality, we refer to the power of hormones as "hormone magic." We believe that the twenty-first century will be the Era of Hormones. It is our earnest desire that people understand the dynamics of hormones, so that these substances, which control so much of the body and mind, can benefit all of us. This goal can be achieved by being aware of how hormones work in our daily lives and utilizing this knowledge to improve our well-being and increase our longevity.

The increase in hormone studies has assisted us in developing a modern understanding of human life. What we are learning through this research is that our basic daily functions, such as running, sweating, and even loving, operate through the intricate work of a variety of hormones. The functions of hormones in the body can be divided into five basic categories:

1. **Growth and Nurture**
   Certain hormones enable a baby to grow into a healthy man or woman.
2. **Procreation and Beauty**
   In order to preserve our species, sexual difference was created; sexual instinct was added; and biological rhythm, including birth, was given to females. An important role of hormones is to maintain appearance and beauty.
3. **Adaptation to the Environment**
   Hormones help maintain homeostasis, or keep the body in harmony with the external factors that influence us. When we face danger, we experience reactions such as an increase in heartbeat and tension in the body. This is due to the function of hormones transmitting information.
4. **Production and Storage of Energy**
   Hormones cause us to have an appetite so that we will consume food. This, in turn, produces energy. Hormones also help store the excess energy as muscle and fat.
5. **Human Intelligence and Emotions**
   Hormones provide us with emotions, intelligence, memory, and creativity. They also give the body the rhythm of work and rest.

Though there are many hormones performing different functions in the body, they all have one purpose in common: to maintain life. I call this system of hormones the "internal body orchestra." Just as numerous different instruments work together in an orchestra to produce beautiful music, our bodies have various hormones working together continuously for an average of eighty-five years, or 2.7 billion seconds, to produce the harmony of life.

The roles and functions of hormones differ tremendously. Some hormones work at maintaining the health of the mind, while others work at resisting illnesses and aging. Some hormones sustain beauty, and others uphold a keen sense of consciousness. This orchestra inside the human body is crucial for each of us to enjoy a good life as a human being.

It has been only in the last one hundred years that the term *hormone* came into common usage. In China and Japan, the term *inner secretions* has been used to refer to hormones. The word "hormone" comes from a Greek word *hormaein*, which means "to set in motion" or "to spur on." This is precisely the function of our hormones: to set in motion the many biological functions that keep us healthy.

At present, we have discovered about eighty different kinds of hormones in the human body. Seven organs, including the brain, adrenal glands, digestive organs, and reproductive organs, secrete some of these hormones. In addition to these organs, blood vessels and human cells produce various hormones as well.

Hormones all work under the basic rule of maintaining homeostasis. This system is designed to keep the body and mind in the best condition possible. We must, therefore, keep a careful balance of hormones in order to maintain good health.

THE INTERNAL BODY ORCHESTRA

The body's hormone balancing is done by the endocrine system, a system made up of glands that produce and send hormones to all parts of the body. The endocrine system and the nervous system perform a similar function: relaying information and commands from the body to the brain, and back to the body again. The nervous system is very quick, usually controlling immediate responses such as the muscle contraction in your leg when you walk. The endocrine system, on the other hand, is much slower and regulates processes, such as metabolism, cell growth, cell aging, and cell death.

Hormones are the messengers that carry information from the brain to every body part. The target cells receive the hormone, which triggers the cell to act in a specific way—to synthesize proteins, replicate, or repair the cell, for example. All of these commands are part of the body's overall response to its surroundings and current situation. Together, your hormones tell your body how to react when you're scared, tired, or ill.

In conjunction with controlling the actions of individual cells, hormones also report back to the various glands, indicating if more or less hormone is needed in the body. This feedback turns off different hormones, keeping them flowing at an optimal level, so that they do not reach a dangerous level.

Recently, hormone researchers have recognized the important symbiotic relationship between hormones and the nervous system, and also between hormones and the immune system. Formerly, it was believed that these three systems operated independently from each other. It is now commonly believed that neurotransmitters, which transmit information in the brain to maintain homeostasis, should actually be viewed as hormones.

Neurotransmitters are the substances used to convey information speedily when our body notices any changes due to stress, illness, or any other factors. Recently, the advancement of brain research has resulted in the discovery of many such transmitters, and we are beginning to see how human emotions actually work. You may be familiar with terms such as *endorphin* or *dopamine*. They are responsible for the various emotions that we feel, such as pleasure, joy, anger, and sadness. Utilizing the basic knowledge of these hormones, many people have tried to create drugs to alter mood. Soon, through hormone research, we will be able to discover what has been shrouded in mystery for centuries.

In our immune system, the substance known as cytokinin should be treated as a hormone as well. It operates much like a hormone but is secreted by the immune cells. Its main role is to allow the immune system to operate. Some of its substances are known as interleukin, or interferon, which can be used to cure liver disease.

Hormones are made up of amino acids or cholesterol, depending on their function. The brain hormone and thyroxin, for example, are made up of amino acids and protein. Protein is able to carry an enormous amount of information. The hormones which use cholesterol as an ingredient are called steroid hormones. These are produced in the adrenal glands, the ovaries, and the testes.

A DELICATE BALANCE

A healthy, well-functioning, and balanced system of hormones prevents infection in the body, fights fatigue and stress, and keeps everything running smoothly. However, a hormone is a delicate substance that operates in minuscule units, measured at only one millionth or one hundred millionth of a milligram. The balance of such small amounts of these powerful substances can easily be upset. The needed amount of hormones secreted by the body is so exact that a small deviation can cause adverse effects in the body and mind.

When any hormone levels are too low or too high, our bodies do not function as they should. We experience damage from hormone imbalance as fatigue, weight gain, loss of enthusiasm and sex drive, and serious illnesses which may include diabetes, coronary heart disease, stroke, cancer, and obesity.

Many aspects of our lifestyle can be responsible for a hormonal imbalance. Hormone levels change when we don't sleep well or eat right, or when we're ill or inactive. The contamination of our atmosphere today is of grave concern because it is affecting the amount of hormones produced in our bodies.

Hormonal imbalance also becomes more of a problem as we age. The older we get, the lower the hormone levels in our bodies become. In fact, these lower levels have traditionally been viewed as a natural part of aging. However, because of recent studies, this view is changing. Many healthcare professionals now believe that our hormone levels don't decline because we age; instead, we age because our hormone levels are declining!

Our careless intake of hormone drugs may also cause an imbalance of the hormone level in our body. An excessive intake of hormones may deprive our body of its ability to naturally produce needed hormones. The side effects of steroid hormones are good examples of this. Artificial and "designer made" hormone tablets sold today may have serious side effects. This gives us cause for concern as hormone tablets gain popularity, often before they have been clinically tested. The delicate balance of hormones is now in serious danger due to misuse.

We need to understand the proper way to utilize hormones so they will benefit us and not cause adverse effects. The correct use of hormones is suitably termed as a "passport to the health and beauty of our body and mind."

HORMONE BALANCING: A THEORY ALREADY IN PRACTICE

Many disorders can now be treated by simply balancing the pertinent hormones, which can be accomplished by supplementing hormones under a doctor's supervision. For more than 40 years, the symptoms of menopause have been treated through estrogen and progesterone supplements. The familiar treatment for diabetes includes replacing the missing or inadequate insulin hormone through regular insulin injections. The potentially debilitating disease of hypothyroidism can be easily treated with a small daily pill. Taking a supplement of the hormone melatonin is a common treatment for certain sleep disorders.

When carried out under the supervision of a doctor, hormone replacement can not only lengthen your telomeres and thereby prolong your life, but it can also improve the quality of life by restoring hormonal balance and allowing your body to function at its best.

We will discuss the benefits of hormone replacement in much greater detail in later chapters. First, however, we will take a closer look at the essential functions of hormones in the brain and body.

The first thing I noticed after about a month was increased energy, and the quality of your life changes because you feel good and you feel good about yourself… You start to carry yourself differently and you want to do things, and you want to get out and enjoy life again.
—Kathy P., patient of the Palm Springs Life Extension Institute

CHAPTER 3

Hormones and Our Emotions

Hormones make us love, make us energetic, and make us attractive. Recent research is unlocking the door into a mysterious region—the will and emotions of humans. What we call the *mind* is made up largely of hormones. More accurately, it is the neurotransmitter which is responsible for how you feel and how your mind works. I am convinced that a thorough knowledge of the brain's inner workings will allow us to develop more potential within ourselves.

We feel diverse emotions every day. For example, you may be in love with someone and feel tremendous happiness. But if that person decides to end the relationship, you feel great pain. When you begin a serious competition with someone, you may feel confident and hopeful. However, if your competitor wins, you feel angry and defeated. These are illustrations of how we can experience a variety of emotions every day.

How many different kinds of emotions do we actually experience? A standard dictionary includes more than one hundred words to describe emotions, including love, joy, anger, sorrow, happiness, depression, melancholy, gladness, pleasure, and fun. How are we capable of experiencing so many complex feelings? The answer lies in the neurotransmitter.

The stage upon which the emotions play is the brain, and the nerves in the brain release the hormone known as the neurotransmitter. Brain cells known as neurons transmit information across the nervous system to other neurons with incredible speed, and neurotransmitters carry this information in much the same way that radio waves transmit information such as sound and images.

The brain has several systems of nerves, which are divided into several groups depending on what information is being sent. The two most important groups are the "A" or "awakening" system nerves, and the "B" or "restraining" system nerves.

A-system nerves secrete hormones such as dopamine and noradrenaline. The function of these hormones is to awaken our senses and activate our feelings. B-system nerves release hormones to counter, or restrain, the awakening or stimulating effects of the A-system hormones. Serotonin is a good example of a B-system hormone. The function of B-system hormones is to calm our heightened senses. The moment the nerve receptor catches the neurotransmitter, a feeling is created. From the hormone researcher's point of view, your mind is created the moment your hormones begin to operate.

DOPAMINE FOR LOVE AND CREATIVITY

Even the way love is born can be explained from the perspective of hormones. Suppose you meet a person you feel attracted to. The meeting of this person will stimulate the A-system nerves in your brain. Synapses, or the protrusions of neurons, will begin to work actively and secrete a large quantity of dopamine, which we call the hormone of joy. Dopamine is then caught by the receptors, and feelings of happiness will begin to move throughout your body.

Dopamine is one of the most important hormones to understand, since it allows us to feel love and creativity. Without dopamine, we cannot experience feelings of pleasure or of being moved. Positive feelings can originate from a variety of experiences, from meeting someone we like to the joys associated with intellectual discovery. We owe it all to dopamine.

Dopamine is absent in the brains of fish. In more highly evolved species, such as mammals, dopamine is used in the areas of movement that utilize the hypothalamus. In humans, the brain cortex secretes dopamine in a large amount, enabling us to express ourselves creatively. This makes the decisive difference between humans and other animals. If you ever find a monkey that can draw a picture, you can be certain that the monkey has an abundant secretion of dopamine.

Dopamine is a truly divine gift. It is so powerful that it can be classified as a stimulant. Using materials broken down from amino acids, the brain produces a variety of substances that would be illegal to buy or sell. Cocaine and LSD are mere imitations of the potent drugs manufactured inside the brain. What our brain produces is more than ten times stronger than the drugs sold on the market.

Imagine that you are walking along the street and see the beautiful scene of cherry trees in full bloom. A-system nerves will produce dopamine, particularly in the area called "A10." You will begin to feel the sensation of joy or even euphoria. You may experience a sharpening of your senses, noticing the rustling of the leaves, stirring air from the gentle breeze, the starry night … you might even be inspired to paint a picture.

Remember those times when you have been moved deeply? Those were the times dopamine filled your brain and awakened your senses, renewed your creativity, and filled your mind with joy and happiness. The American psychologist Maslow mentioned the "Zenith experience" in his writing. A person often starts to move in the direction of success after experiencing something so moving that it cannot even be verbalized. Intense human emotions can elevate our consciousness to a higher level. These emotions can revolutionize our thinking. I call this idea "Dopamine: Rules of Excitement."

Dopamine may be the basic engine that caused humans to evolve. We cannot live as humans without dopamine. I believe dopamine was behind such geniuses as Picasso, Goethe, Mozart, and Edison. Their lives must have been filled with exciting and moving experiences that made them become who they were. Our stressful lives can eventually wear us down so much that our minds and hearts become dull. Cultivating feelings of joy and excitement in your life can revitalize you and bring out your creativity.

There is, however, a problem regarding dopamine. Our brains may be able to produce dopamine in large quantities, but unless there is something to restrain or control that production, the secretion will not cease, and the level of dopamine will be overwhelming. Excessive amounts of dopamine can cause an imbalance in the mind, which can then lead to mental problems of illusion and fantasy. Those suffering from excessive dopamine may not be able to distinguish reality from illusion. The proper or improper amount of dopamine can contribute to one becoming either a genius or a madman.

NORADRENALINE AND THE FIGHTING SPIRIT

In the movie *The Duel at Ganryujima*, Toshiro Mifune played Miyamoto Musashi, who fought with Sasaki Kojiro. The movie depicted the "fighting spirit" that emanated from the two samurai as they faced each other. That fighting spirit is prompted by noradrenaline.

Noradrenaline is related to dopamine, but is far more potent. A-system nerves secrete noradrenaline, especially in the area called "A6." Noradrenaline's toxicity can almost equal the poison in blowfish or poisonous snakes. Of all the substances secreted by the brain, this is the most powerful stimulant. Noradrenaline can also cause severe headaches, trembling, or fainting. These reactions all result from the potency of the hormones released by the brain.

If a person becomes agitated, noradrenaline will serve as a fighting hormone. For example, if a person meets an enemy on the street, the excitement in that instant will cause A-system nerves to transmit the information. Then the A6 system, the largest nerve system in the brain, will release noradrenaline in a large quantity. In addition, noradrenaline can be secreted by the entire nerve system throughout the body and by the adrenal glands as well. This is how noradrenaline can control the entire body in just a split second. This hormone is responsible for our becoming ready for "combat." With this hormone present in our system, our senses become keen, our mind and body prepared for battle. If we could tap into this resource and properly channel this important energy supply for vitality in our life, this hormone would become a tremendous blessing for us. It is truly the source of willpower and courage.

We awake in the morning because noradrenaline is secreted. During the daytime, we can work vigorously because noradrenaline is amply produced. When night comes, the amount secreted lowers, and we become sleepy. Noradrenaline is responsible for keeping our body and mind alert, yet it is also one of the hormones responsible for our restful sleep.

In the midst of our despair and sufferings, noradrenaline will advance to the front line and continue to fight on our behalf even if all others have retreated. Noradrenaline will continue to be produced abundantly in the face of problems for which we have no solutions.

This was illustrated by the following experiment. We put two mice in two boxes, and each box was equipped with a lamp and a buzzer. Every time a lamp went on and a buzzer sounded, an electric current went through the box. Box A was equipped with a button which, when pushed, would prevent the electric shock. In box B, there was no button. The mouse in box A quickly learned to push the button to avoid the electric shock, but the mouse in box B became hopeless and gave up.

The experiment went on for twenty-one hours, and the amount of secreted noradrenaline was measured. The mouse in box A had more noradrenaline than the mouse in box B before it learned how to push the button. Once it learned how to avoid the unpleasant electric shock, the amount of noradrenaline decreased.

From this, we know that noradrenaline continues to flow in our bodies until we solve the problem we are facing. What happens to the noradrenaline that was used and is no longer needed? It will be broken down by decomposition enzymes and diminish as it is washed out through the bloodstream.

THE PROS AND CONS OF ADRENALINE

We occasionally hear about someone who was able to carry incredibly heavy furniture outside when their house was on fire, or someone who jumped astonishingly high to catch a baseball. How could anyone accomplish such incredible feats? A powerful stimulant called adrenaline makes it possible.

Adrenaline is made by noradrenaline, and the two hormones work together like twins. Adrenaline is the hormone released instantaneously when we experience fear or danger; it is a conditional reflex. Adrenaline prepares our body and mind for emergency actions. However, the release of adrenaline is like an explosion, and it does not last. Adrenaline can enable us to accomplish incredible things, but it cannot maintain this ability, and its effects disappear within a few minutes.

Understanding how adrenaline works in your life can be an important asset. Great athletes like golf champion Tiger Woods, baseball player Nagashimo, and champion sumo wrestler Futabayama all mastered their powerful adrenaline.

Golf is said to be a mental sport, since its success does not depend purely upon physical performance. Some of the most important swings that determine a successful outcome are accomplished through mental concentration. If you allow too much adrenaline to flow, the ball will go too far. If the adrenaline is secreted too far in advance of swinging the club, you may miss an important chance to hit the ball. Without an adequate amount of adrenaline, you may find it difficult to concentrate, or you may not be able to exert enough power to hit the ball far.

Most of us do not know how to utilize adrenaline to our benefit. When delivering a public speech, our voice may become too high-pitched, or our throat dry. Our heart rate increases, and it may even become difficult to follow our prepared notes. Most of us can relate to this kind of experience in some way.

The solution is really quite simple. Take a few deep breaths and wait for the rush of adrenaline to pass. Doing some light stretching can help you to calm down sooner and will create more time for productivity. If you are experiencing stage fright and become panic-stricken, you will have even more problems because your adrenaline will pump unrestrained through your body, causing unwelcome reactions.

Adrenaline secretes in the brain as well as in the adrenal glands, and flows through your entire body to fight off stress. If you have to endure stress for too long, your adrenaline increases. If you secrete a large amount of adrenaline, you can develop an aggressive personality. The solution is to discover how your body secretes adrenaline and learn how to stop over-secreting.

You can overcome stress in your life if you know how to use the adrenaline in your body for your benefit. As soon as you feel pressures or stresses, adrenaline begins to be secreted abundantly. Out of many hormones, adrenaline is relatively easy to control. When adrenaline is secreted, it will cause the amount of glucose, which acts as a source of energy, to increase suddenly in the blood. It will awaken our autonomic nervous system to prepare us for either fight or flight. That is why your heart rate increases when you are nervous, and your hands may tremble.

If you begin to understand your adrenaline flow, you will have more confidence in confronting life's many challenges and pressures. If you are out of control and continue to vent your anger, your adrenaline will continue to flow in your system to the point that it will raise your blood pressure and take its toll on your heart and brain. The angry person who continues along this path is actually shortening his life. Do not let adrenaline become your worst enemy.

SEROTONIN

What a great feeling it is to wake in the morning after a good night's rest! After a hard day of work, sleep works wonders in our bodies. It gives us renewed energy to go through another day, refreshing the body and mind.

The substance that induces sleep is a hormone called serotonin. Serotonin is also a source for healing within the body. It can act as a painkiller, and helps stop bleeding.

Serotonin is released by the B-system of restraining nerves to counter the hormones secreted by A-system nerves. When evening comes, noradrenaline begins to decrease, while serotonin begins to increase. The function of serotonin is to regulate dopamine and adrenaline, allowing our bodies to rest. If we were bombarded with "awakening" hormones every day, from morning till night, we would quickly become exhausted.

When we experience a great amount of stress, the serotonin in the brain decreases, sometimes leading to depression. Today it seems that almost everyone, young and old, is complaining about depression. I was in a coffee shop one day and overheard a young lady saying to a friend, "I usually fall asleep all right, but then I wake up in two or three hours and can't go back to sleep. I get so irritable during the day. The doctor told me I have depression. I can't tell my parents, because they'll probably commit me." The young lady seemed to be pleasant and normal, yet she still suffered the effects of depression.

Depression often results from the accumulation of disorders caused by stress, fear, anxiety, and insomnia triggered by a lack of serotonin. Patients suffering from depression show a lower amount of serotonin in the blood. In the past, it was exclusively psychiatrists and psychologists who treated depression, but since the discovery of the connection between serotonin and depression, the illness is now also treated as a hormone disorder.

We are discovering today that low levels of serotonin can cause many other psychological disorders as well, including hypersensitivity to pain, and suicidal or homicidal tendencies.

MELATONIN

Melatonin, another hormone secreted in the brain, leads us into deeper sleep and rest. Airline pilots have often used melatonin to help them with their jet lag. Melatonin is effective and is sold over-the-counter in America without the need for a doctor's prescription. Recent studies of melatonin show that it may delay aging and heighten our immunity. Ongoing research will continue to help us better utilize melatonin, particularly in the area of antiaging medicine. Melatonin will be discussed fully in another chapter.

BETA-ENDORPHIN

Throughout our lives we endure various sorrows and sufferings. We experience sadness when we say farewell to our loved ones or when we suffer a serious illness. As we overcome these episodes, we become stronger. The reason for this inner strength is a group of more than twenty hormones secreted inside the brain that work as anesthetics. The most powerful is beta-endorphin, which is actually internally-made morphine. Beta-endorphin is more than ten times more potent than the morphine that is marketed.

Beta-endorphin works by countering the effects of the "restraining" nerves and their hormones. For example, if you go through a difficult break-up with a partner, the restraining family of nerves becomes active, and you feel a sense of grief and loss. If unchecked, the restraining nerves will continue to increase their release of hormones and will begin to stifle the work of the "awakening" nerves. If you continue in this state for a long period, you may fall into serious depression.

When that happens, beta-endorphin, which is secreted by the pituitary gland in the brain, will counter the restraining nerves and try to revive the awakening nerves. Then the dopamine that was restrained due to grief will begin to secrete, and you will regain your vitality and positive outlook.

Beta-endorphin itself can work as a pleasure hormone as well, prompting such sensations as the euphoria we experience while working on a project that we enjoy.

The basic rule of beta-endorphin is this: when you are in stress, overcome it and get out of it. Every time you overcome stress, you will find yourself becoming stronger.

Beta-endorphin can also affect body development in certain circumstances. We are all familiar with the slender, well-trained body of an accomplished ballerina. For ballerinas, large busts and hips are unnecessary and may even hinder their performances. So how does a ballerina build such a slender and strong body? The answer is beta-endorphin. When a ballerina goes through a vigorous physical regimen every day, beta-endorphin begins to flow in her body far more than normal. She will develop what we call the "beta-endorphin type body."

An excessive amount of beta-endorphin can regulate the secretion of the hormone called LHRH; in other words, it will stifle the secretion of sex hormones. For this reason, a female may miss menstruation, and her breasts and hips will not grow large. In the case of a man, he will notice much less body hair. Beta-endorphin will create a more sexually neutral body and will maintain a body trained for vigorous performances.

The working of the mind is greatly dependent upon the proper working of hormones. The secretions of hormones vary among individuals, and originality and uniqueness of personality emerge partly due to varying degrees of hormone secretion.

Though they are both philharmonic orchestras, there are some differences between the Berlin Philharmonic Orchestra and the Vienna Philharmonic Orchestra. You are the orchestra. You produce your unique music depending upon your individual conductor and the gifted members of the orchestra. Your identity may very well be anchored upon the foundation of your hormone system.

CHAPTER 4

Hormones and a Healthy Body

We have been discussing the neurotransmitters that work in the brain and control our emotions. Now we will explain more about the endocrinal hormones that are secreted by various parts of the body. More than 80 different kinds of hormones regulate our growth, immune system, recovery, and sexuality. Almost all of these hormones are secreted as a result of commands given by the hypothalamus, located inside the brain. The secretions of the endocrinal hormones operate through the following process:

Stimulation Inside and/or Outside the Body

–

Hypothalamus

–

Pituitary Gland

–

Adrenal Gland—Thyroid Gland—Testicles—Ovaries

–

Accessory Thyroid—Pancreas—Digestive Organs—Heart

–

Kidney—Blood Vessels—Immunocyte

First Step: Immediately after receiving stimulation, the hypothalamus sends a command to the pituitary gland.
Second Step: The pituitary gland sends a command to all of the hormone-secreting organs in our body. Our secreting organs then produce the hormones, or regulate the production of the hormones once they have received the command.

This arrangement is similar to the workings of an orchestra. The hypothalamus is the arranger of the music, perfecting its form to create beautiful music. The conductor, who receives this musical score and is responsible for reading it accurately and directing the musicians, is the pituitary gland. Various organs in the body act as musicians, playing their instruments according to the commands of the conductor. In this manner, the symphonic harmony of life continues.

HYPOTHALAMUS: THE ARRANGER OF HORMONES

Many different kinds of hormones are sent to the pituitary gland from the hypothalamus. Let's consider a few of the most important.

Thyrotrophin Releasing Hormone

A person who loses the frontal lobe of his cerebrum loses the ability and will to think. Therefore, we have believed for a long time that the frontal lobe is the center for our motivation.

However, recently we have discovered that the nucleus accumbens of the cerebral limbic system is the source for our motivation. This small organ contains many receptors for the hormones called TRH that are secreted mainly by the hypothalamus. TRH releases the hormone that stimulates the thyroid gland so that it will secrete hormones. As a result, it urges the body to produce thyroid hormones that, in turn, activate cells. It also helps to produce prolactin, a hormone released from the anterior pituitary gland that stimulates milk production after childbirth. TRH stimulates the nucleus accumbens, which produces noradrenaline, the hormone responsible for the fighting spirit.

These hormones serve as receiving antennas. As TRH hormones stimulate the antennas, our brains will "awaken" and our motivation will emerge. When a person becomes depressed and convinces himself that he has no worth, the sharpness of the antenna's receptivity becomes dull. TRH consequently will begin to lower its work performance. On the other hand, if you receive a sincere compliment from your supervisor at work, your antennas will become sharp and TRH will begin to perform well.

How can you create an environment in which TRH can work best? You need ample sleep, because you must sleep well to become awake. TRH will work smoothly if a balance is kept. Disturbances of TRH will follow if you allow the rhythm of rest to become disturbed.

Luteinizing Hormone Releasing Hormone

LHRH regulates our sexuality. LHRH is the most important factor in regulating the menstrual cycle of females. Secreted in 90-minute intervals, it travels to the pituitary gland. It then secretes follicle-stimulating hormones and is transmitted to the ovary, where the follicle is nurtured. The next step is ovulation or fertilization.

Corticotrophin Releasing Hormone

CRH is one of the hormones recently discovered and widely talked about. CRH helps fight stress, increases your ability to learn, and regulates sleep, appetite, and sex drive. CRH stimulates the pituitary gland to secrete the hormone that in turn produces adrenocortical hormones that fight against stress. Recent research has also uncovered a link between CRH and human depression, which may prove to be especially helpful to the increasing older population, many of whom suffer from depression.

Growth Hormone Releasing Hormone

GHRH is responsible for the secretion of *human growth hormone* (HGH). The crucial functions of HGH in childhood and adulthood are discussed in detail throughout in this book.

PITUITARY GLAND: THE CONDUCTOR OF HORMONES

The pituitary gland is a small but important organ attached to the brain that gives direct commands to all the hormone-secreting organs in our body. It can therefore be compared to the conductor of an orchestra. The pituitary gland is divided into two parts: anterior and posterior lobes. The following are some of the hormones secreted by the pituitary gland.

Growth hormones

Growth hormones are produced in children for proper bone and muscle growth until sex hormones kick in. Once the sex hormones are produced and secondary sexual characteristics begin to emerge, the growth hormones are suppressed. Height becomes fixed when the area called the epiphysial line is closed by the secretion of sex hormones. Growth hormones will only secrete enough to maintain the health of bones and muscles, and to maintain various athletic skills.

If a person sexually matures too early, his or her height will be limited. On the other hand, if the initial secretion of sex hormones during puberty is delayed, a person will continue to grow tall. If sex hormones are delayed too long, however, a person may lose the sense of smell and develop color blindness or color weaknesses. This occurs more frequently in men than women.

It is during puberty that height will be determined. Therefore, it is imperative to practice good sleep habits, eat a healthy diet, and exercise to promote a balanced flow of growth hormones during this crucial stage. Growth hormones diminish as we grow older, and this is the primary reason our muscles and bones weaken as we age. Later in this book, we will explore the benefits of replacing growth hormones to regain our energy and youth.

Prolactin

Prolactin is secreted by the pituitary gland and is responsible for breast milk production. It can be called the hormone that is responsible for maternal instinct. After childbirth, this hormone stimulates the milk glands to produce a full breast of milk. Prolactin also stimulates the corpus luteum hormone to oversee the central control of a woman's menstrual cycle. If you look at a newborn baby carefully, you will notice a slight swelling around the baby's nipples. That swelling is the work of prolactin. It contains immune substances produced in the mother's body, and helps develop and organize the breast. We are discovering that this prolactin can be used against stress and to enhance immune capabilities.

Sex hormones

Estrogen, the hormone secreted in the ovary, creates a twenty-eight-day cycle of rhythm in a woman's body, calculating accurately the time of ovulation. The command to secrete estrogen is sent from the anterior lobe of the pituitary gland to the ovary, in the form of a follicle-stimulating hormone.

In men, the pituitary gland gives a command to the testicles to secrete testosterone. The anterior lobe of the pituitary gland is therefore responsible for the ability to engage in sexual activities and reproduction, including production of sperm. The pituitary gland not only gives commands, but also checks and regulates secretion. If something is not secreting properly, the pituitary will urge it to produce more. If it is producing too much, the pituitary will stop it. The pituitary gland possesses elaborate feedback capabilities that keep men functioning.

Vasopressin

The human body is 70 percent water. A healthy person releases about 150 liters of liquid from the kidneys to the renal tube each day. However, the average amount of urine excreted daily is from 1 to 1.5 liters. That means the liquid is concentrated at a ratio of 1 to 100. A hormone called vasopressin is known as an antidiuretic hormone. Its function is to allow the remainder of liquid to be absorbed into our body. If we drink too much liquid, the antidiuretic function cannot keep up. Thus, we will need to go to the bathroom more often. On the other hand, if we sweat a lot and lose the water in our body, then the amount of urine will lessen.

The amount of water in the human body is related to blood pressure, so the vasopressin hormone helps regulate our blood pressure. In conjunction with adrenocorticotropic hormones, vasopressin also promotes memory and learning abilities. Current research is determining how vasopressin could be used for education, as well as how to counter the effects of Alzheimer's disease. We may soon be ready to develop medication to treat senility.

Oxytocin, a hormone for women

This hormone allows the womb to contract, which is an important function during childbirth.

Oxytocin, a peptide (a compound consisting of two or more amino acids) secreted by the hypothalamus, plays a role in social memory. It is often referred to as the "love hormone" because of the part it plays in forging intimate relationships. Oxytocin is released during intimate touch (or even when cuddling) and plays a strong role in maintaining sexual relationships.

HORMONES PRODUCED THROUGHOUT THE BODY

From the hypothalamus to the pituitary gland to the different parts of our body: this is the path information follows through the body by as directed by hormones. We have already discussed the first two steps of endocrinal hormone secretion. The third step involves the various parts of our body that are secreting hormones. Each organ that produces hormones usually produces more than two different kinds. The pituitary gland gives the command as to what kind of hormones to produce.

The Adrenocorticotropic Hormones

The adrenal gland is the fortress for immunity in the body. About the size of the thumb, the adrenal gland is divided into two parts, the cortex and medulla, which sit on top of the right and left kidneys. The adrenal gland produces many valuable and powerful hormones that keep us going. The adrenal cortex in particular secretes hormones that will counter the stresses of the body and mind. This is an essential hormone for our survival. Addison's disease, a disease of the adrenal gland, may leave a person unable to cope with even minor stresses in life. For a victim of Addison's disease, any kind of stress may cause death.

Cortisol is probably the most important adrenocorticotropic hormone for maintaining human life, increasing immunity, and reducing inflammation. It also helps with the metabolism of carbohydrates and proteins, the burning of fat, and the suppression of allergic reactions.

Aldosterone keeps your blood pressure in check. The basic rule for lowering blood pressure is to reduce weight and salt intake. Aldosterone helps regulate the sodium and potassium in our bodies. It works in conjunction with vasopressin to maintain the balance of electrolytes of water, sodium, and potassium.

Dehydroepiandrosterone, also known as DHEA, is the hormone that is secreted more plentifully than any others. DHEA is the hormone recognized as bringing rejuvenation to the human body.

Inside the adrenal gland is an area called the medulla, where adrenaline and noradrenaline are secreted. The hormones produced here work hand-in-hand with those produced in the brain. These hormones increase heart rate, enlarge the arteries, and increase the consumption of oxygen in the heart and muscles. They promote the breakdown of glycogen or fat in the liver, and help blood pressure and blood sugar levels rise to meet the challenges of stress.

In short, the adrenal gland is our defense against stress.

The Source of Vitality and Youth: Thyroid Hormones (T3)

Our body produces power by burning and converting food into energy. The thyroid hormone, secreted by the thyroid gland located above the Adam's apple, is responsible for regulating the production of energy. If there is an excess secretion of thyroid hormones, as in Basedow's disease (also known as Graves' disease), there will be too much energy. The body will be quickly worn out as the "throttle" is wide open for too long. Eating too much kelp, for example, may trigger Basedow's disease because kelp contains a large amount of substances that make up thyroid hormones.

During the heavy bombing of London during World War II, an unusually high number of people in London were affected by Basedow's disease. At the onset of the Gulf War, President Bush was affected by Basedow's disease. The illness also affected Mrs. Bush, and even their dog. Basedow's disease is known as "war disease" because the extreme tension in the face of an enemy's attack may trigger the illness. This is another illustration of how stresses in our life can erode the balance of hormones.

On the other end of the spectrum, if the thyroid is not secreting enough hormone, there will not be enough energy or stamina. This condition is called myxedema (hypothyroidism). The imbalance of thyroid hormones may also be responsible for disorders such as arteriosclerosis, high blood pressure, and senility among people who are not very old.

Among young women, one in twenty to thirty is found to have an abnormality with the thyroid hormone. Basedow's disease, Harshimoto's disease (hypothyroidism), and thyroid cancer are found more often among young women than men. Women are five times more likely to have abnormalities of the thyroid gland. This is because the thyroid gland and female hormones are closely related.

It is reported that among some tribes of American Indians, a bride's neck is measured to indicate how happy she is. Medically speaking, it makes sense to measure the neck for feelings of happiness or euphoria, for the neck may slightly increase in width as the thyroid responds to human feelings, swelling slightly as it produces hormones. Most of the supermodels that our young girls admire tend to be tall and thin, and have long, slender necks. However, if you check the impressionist paintings of beautiful women or the Ukiyoe paintings of Japanese women, you will find women with fuller necks. It seems likely that women with high intelligence, warmth, and friendliness tend to have fuller necks because their thyroid glands are working actively.

Some people born with thyroid glands that do not function properly have been classified as mentally disabled. When given hormone supplements, many have shown remarkable progress. Their eyes become brighter, hair begins to grow, and they look more alert. This kind of treatment has gone beyond the experimental stage and is practiced clinically.

The Gonadotrophic Hormones and Sexuality

There are three important stages in sexual development in the fetus. The first stage is sex determination by chromosomes. A fetus has a total of 46 chromosomes; this set of chromosomes can be either XX or XY. A female is XX, and XY is a male. Immediately after fertilization, however, the fetus behaves as though it wants to become a female.

In the second stage, the gonadotrophic hormones are secreted. During the first eight weeks, the fetus is both male and female, having a "Wolf tube" that is the prototype for the male gonad, and a "Mueller tube" for the female gonad. In ten to twelve weeks, the testes of a male fetus begin to release testosterone, a male hormone, almost like a shower. We have identified this phenomenon recently and have called it "a hormone shower." As a result, from the Wolf tube the male sex organs are created.

If this shower is not adequate, the male organs will not develop properly. If this testosterone shower does not occur at all, as in a female fetus, the Wolf tube will diminish, and the Mueller tube will then develop and create female sex organs.

At the final stage, the genitals are fashioned. It will take almost eighteen weeks for a male fetus to develop male genitals, and almost seven months for his testicles to descend into the scrotum. Compare this to the development of a female fetus, which requires only three months to develop complete female genitals.

Thus, a fetus becomes female in a more straightforward fashion, but a male develops with considerable effort. The average lifespan of a male is also shorter than that of a female. Statistically speaking, an adult male does not possess as much ability to withstand hardships as does a female. Some maintain that the difference is due to the male's XY chromosomes.

There may also be a link between hormonal secretion in the fetus and sexual orientation in adulthood. A study at Juntendo University in Japan showed that pregnant women who were given female hormones instead of corpus luteum hormones to prevent miscarriage in the early stage of their pregnancy gave birth to girls with a high incidence of vaginal cancer, and a high incidence of homosexuality. The secretion of hormones can also be greatly affected by the mental state of the pregnant woman. If a mother undergoes a substantial amount of stress during pregnancy, the fetus may exhibit an abnormal endocrinal secretion of hormones. These findings, combined with the fact that the lack of an adequate hormone shower retards the development of male genitals, demonstrate clearly that hormones have a significant role in sexual development.

During puberty, sexual hormones kick in again and form the secondary sexual characteristics. In boys, the testes begin to produce the cholesterol-based hormone testosterone, as well as sperm. Boys develop more masculine characteristics, such as a beard, a deeper voice, and more muscles. The male secondary sexual characteristics may also include mathematical abilities, aggression, and a desire for power.

Girls, on the other hand, will develop more feminine characteristics with the release of female hormones. The two primary female hormones are estrogen and progesterone. Estrogen is a powerful and essential hormone responsible for developing the female's capacity for pregnancy and childbirth. Incredibly, the amount of estrogen secreted in a woman's lifetime is only one teaspoonful. Estrogen is truly a micro-magician. It works in a woman's body from the onset of menstruation until menopause, without stopping. As long as the ovaries function normally and the menstrual period is regular, estrogen works harmoniously with progesterone.

Inside the ovaries, as a result of the follicle-stimulating hormones, estrogen is created out of a cell called the ovarian follicle. At the early stage of menstruation, this will send signals to LHRH in the pituitary gland to cause ovulation. Without fertilization, the mature follicle will turn into corpus luteum. Then, at the next stage, progesterone is secreted. The body temperature rises as a result, and a woman's rhythmic cycle is maintained. When the amount of progesterone in a woman decreases, it causes what we call PMS, or premenstrual syndrome.

If fertilization occurs, progesterone begins to work overtime, doing important work in the implantation and maintenance of pregnancy. Progesterone will also send signals to stifle sexual desire. Since the female hormones are essential in creating and maintaining female health and beauty, a comprehensive understanding of these hormones is very helpful.

HORMONAL IMBALANCE AND DISEASE

When all the hormones are working together harmoniously, we can enjoy normal development, healthy functioning, and a sense of well-being. However, when there is an imbalance in our hormones, a variety of conditions may develop.

Low Sperm Count

The imbalance of hormonal secretions is one of the major causes of many illnesses peculiar to this day and age. Atmospheric conditions have been altered through pollution. Other environmental factors, such as our water and the food we grow, have a significant impact on mankind. We are beginning to realize that our hormones may be adversely affected by such changes in the environment, and as a result our health may decline.

In 1992, a researcher in Denmark made public the shocking news that among all men in the world, research indicated that sperm count had been reduced by about 50 percent between 1938 and 1990. Researchers cited atmospheric contamination and the prevalence of artificial hormone substances as major causes.

We produce more than one hundred million tons of organic compounds each year. There have been more than one hundred thousand different kinds of chemical substances released into the air, and most of them are enemies to our hormones. An especially harmful substance is dioxin, which is released during trash incineration, because it severely damages gonadal hormones. The damage to gonadal hormones causes a serious imbalance to ovarian hormones in women, while in men it causes a drastic reduction in sperm count.

Some day we may wake up and discover that the average sperm count is hopelessly low. In fact, we have seen an increase in the number of male patients for this very reason. Many of these patients have low sperm counts, and some have a condition known as asthenospermia, or sperm lacking in vitality. It is imperative that we pay close attention to our environment.

Senility

Senility is becoming a social problem in Japan and in the United States as the number of older people increases. Many become forgetful, unable to remember to turn off the stove or recall what they ate for breakfast. Tragically, some cannot even remember the names of their immediate family members. It will be extremely unfortunate if the advancement of medicine allows us to live longer without quality of life.

In the study of senility today, many researchers are looking closely at a hormone that has been linked to Alzheimer's disease: corticotrophin-releasing hormone, or CRH. The function of CRH is to stimulate the adrenal cortex so that it will secrete a hormone called cortisol.

But another important function of CRH has been discovered recently. CRH is found in large numbers in the area of the brain called the hippocampus, which is essential for memory and learning. After age Twenty-five, brain cells begin to die at the rate of two to three per second, which means we lose about ninety thousand cells every day. Because we lose cells in the hippocampus area of the brain, CRH-producing cells are destroyed. If the rate of destruction of CRH cells progresses very rapidly, we call it Alzheimer's disease. When we examine those who are suffering from Alzheimer's disease, we find the number of CRH cells in the hippocampus to be extremely low. Patients also have a lower count of CRH in the brain cortex area.

CRH is made with materials called peptides that can easily dissolve in acid. Therefore, it is quite ineffective to ingest CRH because it will be dissolved by gastric juices before it can be absorbed into one's system. In the United States, researchers have come up with an improved method to orally give CRH to patients without it being destroyed. We may have discovered a solution for curing senility. This is one more example of how important hormone research has become.

Anorexia

Before dying from anorexia, the singer Karen Carpenter had a voice like an angel. Those who mourn her have established a foundation for eating disorders in her memory. Her untimely death brought a new awareness to the world that anorexia is a serious disorder affecting many, particularly young women.

Stress is one of the worst enemies of good health and attractiveness, and it is a formidable opponent of hormones. When our hypothalamus, the center of hormonal secretion inside the brain, undergoes excessive stress, the balance of hormone secretion is adversely affected. Often the adverse effect shows up in the skin. The skin will lose its luster and become grayish due to melanocyte, which is responsible for dark spots on the skin. This melanocyte becomes activated by melanocyte-stimulating hormones that are produced by the pituitary gland. When someone is stressed, the secretion increases, causing the skin to become darker.

Stress also is responsible for lowering the effectiveness of ovarian function, ruining the balance of female hormones, and causing the skin to lose its beauty. Such damage is not confined to the physical body; it will also damage the mind.

Anorexia is a kind of stress-related disorder, as well. The CRH in the hypothalamus increases as stress increases. One of the functions of CRH is to suppress appetite when a person undergoes stress. If stress builds up because of anxiety over body weight, the body will soon refuse to eat, and consequently will suffer from anorexia.

Because of the loss in body weight, a woman's menstruation may cease as her anorexia worsens. Even after she regains body weight, the menstrual cycle may be adversely affected for some time afterward.

If a woman desperately tries to be thin, she must realize the consequences of such efforts. She may attain the goal of thinness, but in the process she may lose her feminine beauty by disrupting the balance of hormones. She may even endanger her life. What does she gain if she loses weight, but loses her health in the process? We must recognize the deleterious consequences of neglecting the rules of hormones.

Aggressive Behavior

One of the most serious problems affecting society today is children tormenting and bullying other children. A child who harasses his peers may be affected by abnormal hormone secretion. In many cases, hormones are behind the antisocial behavior among children around the ages of twelve to fourteen.

The number one suspect is testosterone, the secretion of which increases during puberty. Among male hormones, testosterone is the most powerful. If secreted excessively, it may cause violence. We know that among monkeys, the leader has far more testosterone than any of the other monkeys.

The second suspect is the thyroid hormone. If secreted in the appropriate amount, this hormone increases vitality. But when secreted in an excessive amount, a violent personality can emerge. For example, a child suffering from excess thyroid may utter things that would be unthinkable in a normal situation. He may become impulsive and resort to violence. His heart rate may increase, and his eyeballs may protrude abnormally. If all of these characteristics are displayed, it is fairly certain that the culprit is excessive thyroid hormone.

The third suspect is serotonin. When the secretion decreases, a person may become sensitive to pain or stimulation. He loses control easily and may become violent. The serotonin in our bodies decreases in the evening. Therefore, if a person is more irritable in the evening, excessive serotonin may be the cause.

These hormones may be unbalanced without anyone being aware. The conditions may gradually worsen, until one day the affected child surprises those around him with unpredictable, violent behavior. It is essential to pay close attention to our children each day and observe any slight change in personality. If you notice that your child is unusually irritable, it would be wise to have his hormone levels checked. At a clinic, the test can be conducted easily to determine if your child has a hormonal abnormality. If discovered early, the recovery rate is good. Especially in the case of a thyroid hormone disorder, early detection will assure a 100 percent recovery rate. If serotonin is the culprit, you need to establish a home environment in which the child can receive ample sunlight.

Diabetes

Diabetes is a disorder of metabolism, and results when a deficiency in the insulin hormone, secreted by the pancreas, prevents the energy-giving glucose from ever leaving the bloodstream and entering the cells where it is needed. As a result, glucose that cannot be used builds up in the blood, but the cells still need the energy and call out for more glucose. The liver then releases stored glucose, further raising the blood sugar level. This cycle results in a loss of overall energy, extra strain on the kidneys, weight loss, blurred vision, and frequent infections. In severe, untreated cases, diabetes can be life threatening. Even though the pancreas secretes a proper amount of insulin, the body may not respond properly, which can also cause the disease.

Diabetes is divided into three categories.

Type I, a disease of the autoimmune system, develops in people under age twenty and requires injection of insulin. Some types of viruses that attack the pancreas can cause this type of diabetes.

Type II normally occurs in people over forty and does not necessarily require insulin. This type is called non-insulin dependent diabetes and seems to run in families. More than 30 percent of these patients have a family history of diabetes. Many of them tend to be obese.

Type III includes a variety of conditions. A disorder called acromegalic gigantism is caused by excessive secretion of growth hormone, causing the ends of the limbs to grow larger than normal. Usually this occurs when a tumor develops in the pituitary gland, where growth hormones are secreted. If the tumor develops before puberty, bones will grow excessively and will develop into gigantism. But if it develops after puberty, the tips of the fingers, toes, and chin will grow large. Hyperglycemia is accompanied by diabetes in about 50 percent of the cases. Growth hormone interferes with the work of insulin, and insulin cannot maintain the normal blood sugar level. Type III also includes various disorders connected with Cushing's disease, which is caused by excessive secretion of cortisol. Melanocytoma, which is caused by too much adrenaline or noradrenalin, can also trigger a diabetic condition.

Diet is important for diabetes. If calorie intake is reduced, weight will be lost, and the required amount of insulin will decrease. One must not forget to have enough proteins, fats, vitamins, and minerals, even though the total caloric intake must decrease.

Controlling blood sugar level is the key to controlling diabetes, preventing its progression, and enabling the patient to lead a productive life. The cure requires a tremendous amount of patience and persistence.

High Blood Pressure

Nearly ten million people in Japan, or 8 percent of the population, suffer from high blood pressure. Several factors contribute to this condition: obesity, stress, and too much intake of salt. Surprisingly, hormones could also be the culprit for high blood pressure.

The hormone renin, secreted by the kidney, can raise blood pressure. If the kidney arteries become narrow, the secretion of renin increases. This may be the most prevalent cause of high blood pressure.

The adrenal gland may also secrete an excess of aldosterone. In this instance, aldosterone will keep storing sodium chloride inside our body until the blood vessels become constricted. In many cases, a patient may have a tumor in the adrenal gland, which causes the gland to secrete too much aldosterone. Other symptoms may include excessive thirst, excessive urination, and numbness in the feet and hands. A tumor in the adrenal cortex area may also cause the secretion of too much adrenaline and noradrenalin, which can lead to high blood pressure.

Cushing's syndrome is caused by too much cortisol from the adrenal cortex. This causes high blood pressure and is a hormone-related illness. A patient may develop a red and round face, acne, excess body hair, and a diabetic condition.

One of the symptoms of Basedow's disease is high blood pressure. In this particular case, the maximal pressure could be high, but the minimal pressure could be very low. If a patient with Basedow's disease takes antithyroxin hormone, his blood pressure will return to normal in about two weeks. Sex hormone and growth hormone deficiencies also cause high blood pressure.

Fortunately, today's hormone tests have improved tremendously. All the hormones mentioned here can be checked at a clinic fairly easily, and hormone replacement therapy can then return the hormone levels to a proper balance.

Obesity

Obesity is considered an illness today. Untreated, it can lead to serious conditions such as diabetes, arteriosclerosis, and hyperlipidemia. More recently, we have been seeing a different kind of obesity caused by compulsive eating due to stress.

One hormone works day and night to thwart these dangerous conditions: leptin. Professor Jeffrey Freedman of Rockefeller University first discovered this hormone in fat mice.

When we put on more weight than normal, leptin begins working to suppress the obese tendency, suppressing appetite and expending calories. The hormone was given an appropriate name, *leptin*, which in Greek means *thin*. It has been proven that when a fat mouse is given leptin, his appetite will decrease and his body weight will decrease by 30 percent.

Insulin helps produce this hormone. When we eat, insulin is secreted by the pancreas, which then urges fat cells to produce leptin. Leptin then flows through the blood vessels to the cerebrum, signaling the appetite-control center in the hypothalamus, and appetite drops. This is why we feel full after we eat. Leptin will also try to burn any excess fat that we consume. This entire phenomenon is the work of the hormone leptin, which is dedicated to homeostasis, or balance.

When we take in more fat than leptin can get rid of, we gain weight. We live in a society characterized by overindulgence and easily end up eating far more than our body requires, and even leptin cannot reverse the effect.

Since discovering leptin, we are looking at the "fat cells" from a new perspective. We have always considered the fat cell a villain. However, when you lose weight suddenly, you will experience a temporary interruption of your body rhythm because of the loss of a protein called "compliment," which is secreted by fat cells.

Since the discovery of leptin, a remarkable diet hormone, our thinking concerning diet and obesity has changed dramatically. We may now be within reach of a diet pill that really works.

Impotence

Impotence is a condition many men begin to secretly worry about when they reach andropause (or "male menopause," a condition with menopause-like symptoms; more about andropause later in the book). Some of those suffering from impotence buy expensive "tonics" or go through stress-reduction counseling sessions. However, in some cases of impotence, the cause may be a condition called High Prolactin Disorder, which results from a tumor on the pituitary gland in the brain. The tumor produces an excess amount of a hormone called prolactin, which in women normally urges the mammary gland to produce milk. If it is secreted in excess in men, it will suppress male hormones and cause impotence.

This tumor is rather difficult to detect at first. Once it becomes large, a man may find that his nipples secrete. He may experience headaches due to the oppression of the optical nerves by the tumor, and a narrowing in his field of vision. Once detected, the tumor can be removed through the nose. After the tumor is removed from the pituitary gland, impotence is quickly cured after only a few days. Because it is not malignant, it can also be treated with a medicine called bromocryptin if it is discovered early.

Hormone Receptor Disorders

Other kinds of hormone disorders are associated with the hormone receptor. We are discovering more and more hormonal disorders even occurring in cases when the secretion level is normal. These are typically related to problems with receptors.

A hormone called Beta 3 adrenaline helps break down the fat stored in our body, or burns the unnecessary fat cells. Obesity can develop when there is an abnormality in the amino acids of this hormone's receptor. In Japan, new research indicates that 1 in 3 people has an abnormality in the receptor. You can have your receptor checked at your nearest clinic.

Some people never gain weight though they eat all the time. Others eat little and yet gain weight. We have assumed this is because of the difference in metabolism. As research reveals new findings about Beta 3 adrenaline, however, our thinking about obesity has changed dramatically.

Those with an abnormality in receptors for Beta 3 adrenaline burn two hundred fewer calories per day than a person with normal receptors. If you have the abnormality, you must try to reduce your food intake by two hundred calories.

New research indicates that the number of hormone receptors also determines one's height. In the past, we assumed that height differences resulted from the difference in the secretion of growth hormones. We believed that if the pituitary secreted a small amount of growth hormones, no matter how many nutrients were ingested, height would not increase.

As hormone studies have progressed, we have come to understand that it is the number of hormone receptors that determines height. This was first discovered by the research group led by Dr. David Golde at the Memorial Sloan-Kettering Cancer Center in the United States. Their research has clearly revealed the relationship between the number of receptors and height. In comparing the white blood corpuscles of pygmies in Africa and those of hereditarily tall Americans, they discovered that the pygmies had only one-tenth the number of receptors as the average hereditarily tall person.

This receptor for the growth hormone is called IGF-1 and is produced in the liver. IGF-1 is secreted abundantly during childhood and puberty. It mediates the work of growth hormones and urges the growth of bones. It can exert its power only when the antenna of the receptor catches its power. Therefore, if the number of receptors is limited, so is its power.

What causes the low number of antennas in this receptor? Research indicates that among those who are hereditarily short, white blood corpuscles lack the ability to "copy" the genetic information for creating receptors for the hormone. Therefore, the number of receptors is genetically suppressed.

Understanding our hormone levels is essential in maintaining good health and preventing disease. For self-tests that may help you determine your hormone type, please see Appendix A.

CHAPTER 5

The Disease of Aging

We have discussed the essential role of hormones in health, beauty, and emotional well-being, and the necessity of a careful balance of these hormones. Unfortunately, our hormone levels begin dropping from about age twenty-five or thirty, just as our telomeres begin to show signs of serious decline. For most of us, the effects of this decline are so subtle we don't notice them until we're in our forties or fifties. This is when we begin to realize that even if we live a healthy lifestyle, we don't have as much energy as we used to, we're putting on weight, beginning to go gray, and discovering wrinkles on previously smooth skin. These are all outward signs of a weakened or imbalanced hormone system, and the onset of the disease called aging.

Other signs include thinning skin, a less-efficient metabolism, and brittle bones. Our weakened systems are caused by insufficient hormone levels in the body and their effect on our telomeres, the part of the chromosome that tells the cell to keep regenerating. Hormone deficiency also weakens the organs, raises the level of triglycerides and

LDL (bad) cholesterol, lowers the levels of HDL (good) cholesterol, and increases the chances for illness and disease.

Aging is a syndrome controlled by the inborn process of progressive tissue degeneration, a neuroendocrine clock that gradually diminishes hormone levels and reduces the capacity of DNA to repair itself. Although aging is not yet recognized as a disease by the Food and Drug Administration (FDA), the US Patent Office, or some of the medical community, it has the earmarks of disease: "Progressive disability leading to death, with no cure." It is particularly interesting that human beings who die of old age do so at different chronological ages, because their biological ages can vary greatly.

HOW OLD ARE YOU REALLY?

There is a difference between how long you have been alive and how old you are. When you were born, the hospital issued a birth certificate listing your name, parents, and date of birth. Many people believe that this date of birth determines their age. However, this number merely tells you how many years you've been alive and is not an accurate measure of your health, or how much your cells and organs have deteriorated.

So instead of simply prescribing a treatment based on a person's chronological age, which is determined by date of birth, enlightened practitioners first determine how old an individual is biologically. For example, a twenty-year-old, because of illness or injury, could have a biological age somewhere in his or her fifties, and an active fifty-year-old may test biologically in his or her mid-thirties.

DETERMINING BIOLOGICAL AGE

With recent advances in research, we believe we can reverse many of the symptoms of aging. But before we can prove the possibility of life extension, we must first prove that a given therapy is reversing biological age. Currently, the only other way to determine the efficacy of any longevity or antiaging treatment regimen is to wait fifty to one hundred years and then evaluate the results retrospectively. This method is very impractical for those of us who want to do something now about our health and the aging process.

Therefore, we have developed a means of evaluating potential life-extending treatment methods over a short period of time, in the two- to five-year range. These tests measure biological age so we can determine whether a patient is biologically growing younger as a result of antiaging therapy, or is continuing to age. This helps us evaluate which antiaging regimens are effective.

How do we determine an individual's biological age? Eventually, telomere testing may give us more clues to biological age, but this type of testing is not yet widely available and is not system- or organ-specific. The most reliable tests for biological aging that are currently available fall into two basic categories. The first deals with the body's ability to function actively, including forced vital capacity, or lung function, and cardiac and renal functions. The second category is based on the cellular or molecular changes in the body, including bone loss, fingernail growth, change in percentage of lean body muscle, declining levels of various hormones, sensory and neurologic deficits, and decreasing immune function.

The following is a brief overview of the methods used to determine biological age.

Forced Vital Capacity

It is well-documented that forced vital capacity, or the amount of air a person can expel in one second, changes with age. A twenty-year mortality study showed that death related predictably to a biannual measured forced vital capacity. Excess mortality directly related to poor lung function was noted in the elderly, as well as in the young, in both sexes, and in nonsmokers as well as smokers. The decreased forced vital capacity could be the result of loss of muscle power or a stiffer, less compliant chest wall or diaphragm.

Measuring Muscle Mass and Function, and Body Fat

Aging is also associated with decreased muscle function and mass. This causes a decrease in hand grip strength and decreased physical endurance and physical capacity. Hand grip strength can be measured easily by a dynamometer, and muscle functions of different extremities can be measured by isokinetic computerized machines.

Age is also associated with an increase in percentage of body fat. This change can be measured by skin calipers, skin impedance measurements, and the water immersion method.

Cardiac Function

It has been known for many years that aging is directly related to decreased resting cardiac output. Cardiac function can be determined by cardiac hemodynamic studies conducted in a cardiologist's office.

Renal (Kidney) Function

Progressive decline in renal function is also associated with age and begins essentially in the middle of the fourth decade. This can be documented by a kidney creatinine clearance (filtration) test.

Bone Loss

Bone loss is a significant problem that accompanies aging, leading to skeletal collapse and fractures. This is the leading cause of disability in elderly women. Bone loss changes can be documented by a radioisotope bone scan, which is easily performed in most hospital radiology departments.

Fingernail Growth

Studies have shown that the rate of fingernail growth, measured over one year, can give quantifiable information when correlated with age. Linear nail growth decreases 50 percent over a person's life span. Changes in fingernail growth rate can be measured by marking the fingernail.

Neurologic Function

Decreases in neurological function may also be noticed with increased age. These functions include hearing, sight, reaction time, and memory, and can be measured individually by a physician in an office setting.

Skin Changes

The skin also undergoes changes with age. This can be measured by a skin biopsy or skin turgor test. Skin turgor is measured by pulling up the skin on the back of the hand and observing the time it takes for the skin to return to its natural position.

Endocrine System Hormone Levels

There are many hormones that decline with age. Some decline in a linear fashion, while others do not. Of the various hormones, dehydroepiandrosterone (DHEA) and melatonin decline in the most linear fashion (almost in a straight line) beginning in the second decade. Therefore, the DHEA hormone (produced by the adrenal gland) and the melatonin hormone (produced by the pineal gland) are the most accurate in predicting biological age. Other hormones that decline with age are human growth hormone, the sex hormones such as testosterone, estrogen, and progesterone, and sometimes thyroid hormones.

Aerobic Capacity

Aerobic capacity has long been shown to decline with age. Measuring aerobic capacity involves measuring the energy that is expended to go a certain distance or perform a certain physical feat.

Immunicological System

Immune responses decrease in the elderly such that skin allergy test responses are reduced significantly. This can be tested by measuring the reaction to a tuberculin or tetanus skin test. Human cytokine production also declines with age in that interleukin-s decreases with age, whereas interleukin-3, -4, and -10 increase with age. The B-lymphocyte cells, monocytes, and macrophages remain unchanged with age; however, the number of T-cell lymphocytes and natural killing cells (NK cells) also decrease with age, particularly the CD3, CD4, and CD8 cells. Not only the number, but the response of T-cells also decreases with age. There is a marked age-related decline in human IgG antibodies and a less marked decline in IgM antibodies beginning at age sixty. This is another reason why people over sixty are much more susceptible to infection.

All these changes in the immune system can be tested and assessed to help determine biological age.

FOLLOW-UP TESTING

Once we have determined biological age, subsequent tests can tell us how quickly a person is aging. More importantly for us, biological age gives us a standard by which we can measure progress as an individual goes through treatment and grows younger. Biological age determinants are a quick and accurate description of how the body responds to any antiaging treatment. Waiting fifty years to see the results of longevity therapy is simply not necessary.

A sample prescription for biological age tests that can be performed at any local hospital is included in Appendix B. If you would like to have these tests done, please call the Palm Springs Life Extension Institute for no-obligation information.

BIOLOGICAL AGE TESTING IN PRACTICE

Here is how biological age testing works in a clinical setting.

A forty-seven-year-old patient with two years of hormone replacement therapy at the Palm Springs Life Extension Institute underwent a complete panel of biological aging tests in twelve biological age, health, and fitness areas, including lung capacity, memory, and reaction time. The patient had an average tested biological age of thirty-seven years, ten years younger than her chronological age. Of her twelve scores, seven were more typical of women in their twenties.

Her test results were useful to her, not only to confirm the wisdom of her health choices, but also to help her determine the areas that had improved most and those that still needed work. Aside from feeling and looking good, she now has measurable evidence that she has turned back the clock—in this case ten years!

YOU DON'T NEED TO WAIT ANY LONGER

At the Palm Springs Life Extension Institute, we offer treatment results today. We believe that a young body is a healthy body, so we are dedicated to keeping the body as young as possible. To do this, we have put the theories about telomerase and hormone replacement into practice. Our clientele numbers more than 2,500, and because of this very large research base, we don't have to wait fifty years to see the outcome of total hormone gene therapy. We are seeing, testing, and measuring it today.

CHAPTER 6

The Master Hormone

After a certain age, lifestyle alterations alone are not sufficient to keep hormones at optimal levels and our telomere tips consequently long and youthful. Once on a program of balanced hormone replacement therapy, people who are considered senior citizens have as much energy and drive as twenty-five-year-olds. Their libidos have returned, wrinkles and gray hair have faded, fat is lost and muscle is taking its place, the diseases associated with aging are disappearing, and they have a new, upbeat outlook on life. They seem to have been able to stop the aging process, and in some cases reverse it, simply by refueling their bodies with the essential elements of a balanced hormone gene therapy, which we will outline.

One prominent part of this therapy is a powerful, almost magical, hormone recently identified by researchers as a key to youth and health: human growth hormone, or HGH. Many of the functions of HGH, and the cycles of HGH release, are surprisingly parallel to those of telomerase. As HGH levels decline, so do those of telomerase. As we learn more about its relationship to the organs and cells of the body, and especially to telomerase, HGH may well prove to be one of the most important and powerful substances in the human body.

HGH controls the body's overall growth, and was originally thought to be important only during the formative, adolescent years when the body changes and grows very rapidly. After this initial period of growth, it was assumed that HGH levels dropped because the hormone was no longer needed. However, it is now clear that HGH plays a vital role in maintaining the health of the body.

HGH is a protein hormone that affects all endocrine glands and influences the growth and development of nearly every organ and tissue in the body. HGH regulates the body's metabolism of proteins, electrolytes, and carbohydrates, and controls how the body uses fat. Given that HGH influences nearly all hormones, perhaps the strangely coincidental cycles of HGH and telomerase are not so coincidental at all.

HGH is secreted by the somotropic cells of the anterior lobe of the pituitary gland, located at the base of the brain. Because it originates in the somotropic cells, HGH is also known internationally by the name somatotropin. For the purposes of this book, however, we will continue to refer to it as human growth hormone, or HGH.

HGH RELEASE

HGH differs from many of the other hormones in the way it is secreted from the pituitary gland. Some hormones are secreted at a constant rate. In the case of HGH, however, research has indicated that while the pituitary gland typically releases HGH in small quantities throughout the day, by far the major secretion occurs at night, peaking one to two hours after the onset of deep, rapid eye movement (REM) sleep. This is a much higher peak than is ever reached during the day or even during exercise.

The output of HGH is regulated by two other hormones produced by the hypothalamus: the growth hormone releasing hormone (GHRH) and the growth hormone inhibiting hormone (GHIH). Research has shown that GHRH pulses at regular intervals throughout the day, in a pattern that does not match the secretion of HGH. However, GHIH, normally present in high amounts, occasionally drops to low levels, allowing the release of HGH into the bloodstream. So GHIH is the true gatekeeper of HGH. When GHRH and GHIH are in balance, the body produces, releases, and uses exactly the amount of HGH that it needs. Acromegaly, or gigantism, can result from too much HGH in the body.

Factors that can increase the amount of HGH in the body are:

Physiological

- Deep Sleep
- Strenuous Exercise
- Stress Conditions
- Protein Ingestion
- Fasting
- Hypoglycemia

Pharmacological

- Insulin with Hypoglycemia
- Post Glucagon
- HGH Releasing Hormone
- Estrogen
- Peptides (hexarelin)
- Melatonin
- Potassium I.V.
- Amino Acids

Diseases

- Starvation and Anorexia Nervosa

MEASURING HGH

HGH is released into the bloodstream in only minute amounts during the day, and the nighttime peak lasts for a very short period of time. The levels drop again as fast as they shoot up, and then seem to virtually disappear. This feature of HGH secretion makes it difficult to measure HGH levels; we would have to know the precise moment HGH was being released in order to directly and accurately measure for appropriate amounts. To get an exact idea of a body's HGH level, we can test for a product that rises and falls with HGH levels. In this case, that product is insulin-like growth factor-1(IGF-1).

IGF-1, also called somatomedin C, is a protein produced in the liver by HGH. IGF-1 binds to cells and carries out its growth-promoting and regenerating duties. There is a link between the levels of IGF-1 and HGH, but IGF-1 levels in the body are much more constant, and therefore easier to measure, than HGH. By testing the IGF-1 levels, we can get an estimate of how much HGH the body is secreting.

So what does it mean if our IGF-1 levels, and therefore our HGH levels, are low?

OUR NEED FOR HGH

For more than fifty years, HGH has been used almost exclusively to counter the effects of hypopituitary disease in children. When the pituitary gland fails to produce enough HGH, a child's growth is stunted, resulting in dwarfism. In children with normal pituitary gland production, HGH tells the body when and how much to grow. So just like telomerase, HGH levels are highest during the early years, when the body is growing quickly. Because HGH release is related to sleep, adolescents will often need more sleep to bring HGH levels to their necessary peak. Release patterns also explain why we feel so sluggish and tired when we haven't slept well. If we never get to the REM stage of sleep, or don't stay there long enough, we may not get all of the HGH we need to function during the day.

But after adolescence, when we've grown as tall as we're going to, is the need for HGH over? Our bodies seem programmed to think so. Once the big push to get our adolescent bodies to grow is passed, our HGH levels continually decrease every year. Humans under age twenty-one have high HGH levels and low GHIH levels. This promotes continued growth and overall health. As we age, however, the levels of GHIH climb and stabilize at high levels, which do not allow HGH into the bloodstream on a regular basis. In fact, studies show that by age forty, our HGH levels are at only 40 percent of what they were at age twenty. The rate of decline is continuous, and in another forty years, at age eighty, our HGH levels drop to only 5 percent of the twenty-year-old level.[9]

HGH DEFICIENCY

For years, heath care professionals have considered this drop in HGH levels to be a normal and expected part of aging. In response to complaints about lack of energy, initiative, and physical strength, doctors have conventionally said, "What do you expect? You're not as young as you used to be."

But recently, connections have been made between certain health conditions and the decline in HGH levels. A drop in levels is directly linked to an increase in total weight and body

---

9 Hertoghe T. "Growth Hormone Therapy in Aging Adults." 1996 Annual Conference on Antiaging Medicine and Biomedical Technology, Las Vegas, Nevada.

fat, decrease in muscle mass, decreased bone mass and strength, reduced exercise capacity, and an overall decrease in energy. Low HGH levels are also associated with an increased risk of cardiovascular disease, reduced life expectancy, weakened immune system, dry skin, cold intolerance, reduced basal metabolic rate, sleep dysfunction, lower HDL (good) cholesterol, an inability to concentrate, impaired memory, and irritability.[10] In rare cases, low levels of HGH can lead to dwarfism.

Factors that cause HGH levels in the body to decrease are:

Physiological

- Hyperglycemia

Pharmacological

- Somatostatin
- Cortisol

Diseases

- Obesity
- Thyroid Disease

In recent years, the medical world has finally started to recognize and accept aging as a disease and has begun to treat the worldwide epidemic of Adult Growth Hormone Deficiency. The existence of so many typical symptoms qualifies HGH deficiency as a disorder, or a clinical syndrome, just as HGH deficiency is a recognized disease in children.

We can also now view aging as a disease because we have discovered its cause. We know that it is caused, at least in part, by declining hormone levels and an HGH deficiency. By all modern medical standards and ethics, it makes absolutely no sense to sit by and let nature take its course, doing nothing to stop the physical deterioration that comes with age. Indeed, we already

10 Meling TR, Nylen ES. "Growth hormone deficiency in adults: a review." *Am J Med Sci* 311(4):153–166, Apr 1996.

accept medical intervention for many of the individual symptoms. It would be unthinkable to withhold treatment for heart disease, arthritis, diabetes, cataracts, or cancer. And yet these are often just symptoms of the larger disease we call aging. Instead of treating one symptom after another, wouldn't it be better to simply treat the disease that was causing the symptoms in the first place?

WHERE WE GET HUMAN GROWTH HORMONE

So why, with all these incredible benefits, has it taken so long for HGH to become available for adult use? The main reason is that until recently, HGH was very hard to come by. HGH is a complex chain of 191 amino acids curled up like a rattlesnake, and it could not be synthesized as easily as some of the more common hormones such as DHEA and estrogen, which are cholesterol based. HGH is also species specific, meaning that the growth hormone found in animals will not work as a substitute in hormone-deficient humans.

For years, the only source for HGH was the pituitary glands of human cadavers, which made the supply scarce. This scarcity limited its use to the treatment of children with an HGH deficiency, who would otherwise not achieve normal height or development.

In addition to its scarcity, this method of harvesting HGH was not 100 percent safe. Patients in HGH replacement therapy using HGH from cadavers showed an increase in the incidence of Creutzfeldt-Jakob Syndrome, or Mad Cow Disease, which is an infectious viral disease that is typically fatal. This frightening aspect scared many researchers away from even studying HGH replacement.

Eventually, researchers uncovered the secrets of synthesizing HGH, and, at least in the United States, cadaver HGH was banned. Unfortunately, there are still those who, because of incomplete or incorrect information, have trouble accepting this fact. Red Cross workers have been known to refuse blood donated by adults who are undergoing HGH replacement.

Biosynthetic HGH was made possible only by the advent of recombinant DNA technology. HGH is often referred to as recombinant HGH (rHGH), but because it is now the only source of HGH, most have dropped rHGH in favor of the simpler HGH. Because we no longer get this precious substance from cadavers, the threat of disease from the hormone is now completely absent.

Recombinant DNA technology uses the DNA from a cell of human growth hormone and puts it into another cell (usually E-coli cells or human breast cells) that will divide and reproduce quickly. The result is a large supply of cells that are identical in every way to a healthy growth hormone cell, such as those you would find in your pituitary gland. The manufactured cell is an exact twin because recombinant HGH is duplicated from the genetic blueprint of the HGH that is already in your body.

Because it is identical, recombinant HGH will not cause any disease, discomfort, or unpleasant side effects. It's like drinking water. Water makes up about 60 percent of our body mass. When we drink more water, our body accepts it because it is molecularly identical to the water we already have in our system. It doesn't matter if the water came from a bottle or from your kitchen sink.

The development of recombinant technology opened the door and paved the way for the groundbreaking research that is the basis for this book. With this research, the technology and professional know-how to use it, and the safe and increasingly inexpensive recombinant HGH, everything is now in place to help you win the war against aging.

EARLY HGH STUDIES

The first study using hormones to combat the symptoms of aging was conducted in the late 1960s by the Russian gerontologist Vladmir Dillman. His research provided evidence that we begin aging in our twenties, at the same time our HGH production levels fall. Many more studies since then have furthered our understanding of the essential role hormones play in helping keep the body rejuvenated.

One of the first studies conducted replenishing adult HGH was performed by Dr. Jorgensen of Copenhagen in 1989. He administered HGH to adults in a carefully monitored, double-blind, placebo-controlled crossover study. The purpose of the study was to evaluate the benefits of HGH replacement therapy in adults who had experienced a loss of muscle volume, strength, and exercise capacity—all considered a natural part of the aging process.

Jorgensen found that on all three counts, there was a marked improvement. Isometric strength and exercise capacity increased, as did the mean muscle volume of the thigh. The total body weight remained the same, however, because the amount of fatty tissue decreased in proportion to the muscle gain.[11]

A study in 1989 by Dr. F. Salomon also reported similar significant benefits from HGH therapy. Salomon and his colleagues administered HGH to twenty-four HGH-deficient adults and observed increases in the body's metabolism and lean body mass, as well as a decrease in body fat.[12]

---

11 Jorgensen JO, Pedersen SA, et al. "Beneficial effects of growth hormone treatment in GH-deficient adults." *Lancet* 1(8649):1221–1225, 3 Jun 1989.

12 Salomon F, Cuneo RC, Hesp R, et al. "The effects of treatment with recombinant human growth hormone on body composition and metabolism in adults with growth hormone deficiency." *N Eng J Med* 321:1797–1703, 28 Dec 1989.

But the most promising research in HGH replacement for adults came from Dr. Daniel Rudman of the Medical College of Wisconsin. Rudman is considered the pioneer in HGH replacement research, and ever since his study on the effects of HGH replacement in aging men was published in the *New England Journal of Medicine* in 1990, doctors and patients alike have been eager to learn even more about this amazing hormone.

For many years, Dr. Rudman had been asking these questions: "Do hormone levels control the aging process? If they do, then does replacing the hormone levels to the youthful range in humans reverse the effects of aging?" Dr. Rudman conducted his study on twenty-six men from a nearby Veterans Administration hospital, ranging in age from sixty-one through eighty. These men were considered to be in good health for their age, but they all had low levels of HGH.

At the end of only six months of treatment with HGH, the results were amazing. Dr. Rudman reported that the men who received HGH experienced an increase in lean body mass and a decrease of up to 14 percent in overall body fat. These men also showed a greater lumbar bone density and thickened skin. Dr. Rudman's conclusion was that the negative side effects usually associated with aging (weaker muscles, higher fat content, thinning bones) are caused, at least in part, by an HGH deficiency. Even more promising was his report that these side effects could be stopped, and in some cases the damage undone, by replacing the HGH. The restoration of skin thickness and bone mass showed this reversing effect. Dr. Rudman said, "The effects of six months of HGH on lean body mass and adipose-tissue mass were equivalent in magnitude to the changes incurred during ten to twenty years of aging."[13]

13 Rudman D, et al. "Effects of human growth hormone in men over 60 years old." *N Eng J Med* 323:1–6, 1990.

Imagine HGH taking only six months to repair the damage done in a decade of aging. Dr. Rudman's study excited keen interest in the general population, the medical community, and in other researchers, and paved the way for continuing research, which has proven that growing young is no longer a fantasy—it is today's reality.

THE NEXT WAVE

After examining various studies published between 1990 and 1992 showing HGH's ability to reverse changes associated with aging, Stanford University medical researchers wrote a review that concluded, "It is possible that physiologic HGH replacement therapy might reverse or prevent some of the inevitable sequela of aging." Stanford was referring to studies showing that HGH can restore youth and health in the following ways:

- Decrease the percentage of body fat while increasing lean muscle mass by stimulating the body's ability to increase protein synthesis.
- Increase bone mass, reversing damage that leads to osteoporosis.
- Reverse the degeneration of neurological functions.
- Improve cardiac function.
- Improve skin tone, thickness, and elasticity.
- Improve pulmonary functions.
- Improve the functioning of the immune system.
- Improve kidney function.
- Improve exercise and aerobic capacity and endurance.
- Help wounds heal faster.
- Improve cartilage synthesis for stronger joints.

- Reverse the normal, age-related shrinkage of organs like the liver and spleen.
- Increase basal body temperature rates.
- Decrease levels of cholesterol.
- Stimulate the body's ability to transport and absorb amino acids and other essential nutrients.
- Affect the endocrine glands and influence growth.
- Rejuvenate sex drive.

These studies show that HGH has clearly earned its place as the master hormone because it affects all the other hormones and organs throughout the body. And while hormones such as melatonin and DHEA affect the entire body as well, the effects of HGH are much more powerful and dramatic and become evident much more quickly. HGH also has unsurpassed reparative and restorative powers that can reverse damage and even regrow failing organs—something no other hormone can do.

THE LATEST RESEARCH

In most recently published studies, HGH continues to live up to the reputation it garnered from earlier studies. In addition, HGH has been confirmed as one of the few effective, long-term treatments for heart failure patients, has resulted in better recovery in burn and surgical patients, successfully treated life-threatening malnutrition in kidney-failure patients, aided post-menopausal women trying to shed pounds or build stronger bones, been recommended for its wound healing, and been noted to improve sexual function.

For those who take HGH on a regular basis, research reported in the past year confirms a wide variety of long-term benefits, including improved general well-being, higher energy levels, a more positive emotional outlook, the ability to sleep better, better body composition, a more efficient metabolism, and a reduction of days spent in a hospital or missed from work.[14]

In London's St. Thomas Hospital, researchers reported that growth hormone replacement will probably become standard therapy for growth hormone-deficient adults in the near future. They based this conclusion on studies showing that HGH is well tolerated, restores lean body and bone mass, reduces fat mass, increases total body water, increases exercise capacity and protein synthesis, makes favorable changes in plasma lipids, and improves the quality of life and psychological well-being.[15]

TOMORROW'S RESEARCH

The National Institute on Aging, as well as medical centers and research institutes around the world, are currently funding research into the effects of HGH replacement in adults. While its efficacy is no longer a question, the medical community wants to know exactly how and why HGH works. The telomere and telomerase connection is also high on the list of research projects. But while scientists research these links and details, we have the research base and the experience to safely and effectively use the power of HGH now.

THE AUTHOR'S STORY: DR. CHEIN AND THE PALM SPRINGS LIFE EXTENSION INSTITUTE

I became interested in hormone replacement therapy when I worked in physical medicine and rehabilitation with patients

---

14 Verhelst J, Abs R, et al. "Two years of replacement therapy in adults with growth hormone deficiency." *Clin Endocrinol (Oxf)* 47(4):485–494, 1997.

15 Christ ER, Carroll PV, et al. "The consequences of growth hormone deficiency in adulthood, and the effects of growth hormone replacement." *Schweiz Med Wochenschr* 127(35): 1440–1449, 1997.

recovering from injuries that had damaged various glands. In patients whose damage required hormone replacement, there was a rapid improvement as soon they were treated with hormone therapy. They quickly recovered lost energy, stamina, and muscle strength.

Since hormone replacement worked so well for these patients, I began to wonder what it might do for me. At age forty-two, I had begun suffering angina pains, my cholesterol and triglyceride levels were up, and I was gaining weight. In short, I was aging, I was in pain, and my cardiologist warned me to cut back on work or risk devastating health problems.

Other hormones such as melatonin and DHEA had been shown to slow aging, but nothing had been shown to *reverse* aging until Dr. Rudman showed that HGH could accomplish this. I decided to try total hormone gene therapy on myself. I wanted to replace all my hormones to the levels of a twenty-year-old and see if I could reverse my biological age. My theory was that if I could restore my young adult hormone levels, then I shouldn't have any more symptoms, since I hadn't had any of these problems when I was twenty. My cholesterol and triglycerides should come down, and my chest pains should go away.

Not surprisingly, my lab results showed that many of my hormones were severely deficient, some falling off the reference range for normal adults in my age group. Within six months of replacing my hormones, my chest pains stopped, my cholesterol and triglycerides became normal, and I started losing my big belly. The results were amazing both to me and my doctor.

In 1994, I opened the Palm Springs Life Extension Institute, which functions under the belief that total hormone gene therapy is the best option open to us today to prevent the disease of aging.

PRACTICING MEDICINE THE RIGHT WAY

The current state of medicine is to wait until you are sick before going to a doctor. The doctor then diagnoses your illness and treats you. Once you recover, you don't see your doctor again until another infirmity strikes you.

This cycle is totally wrong. What should happen is this: you see your doctor when you are well and let him or her prescribe a course of action to keep you well. This approach costs less than curing an illness, and the patient is much better off in the long run.

That is what we do at the Palm Springs Life Extension Institute. We prescribe a treatment plan designed to try to prevent the disease of aging.

CHAPTER 7

HGH for Growth and Maintenance

THE BIG PICTURE

We have talked about what HGH is and where we get it. We have also briefly discussed some of the research that has been done on growth hormone. We can now combine growth hormone replacement studies with our data from the Palm Springs Life Extension Institute to get a much better picture of how dramatic and powerful HGH is, and exactly how it is used in the body.

To understand more about how HGH works in the body, we can compare it to the effect of a puppeteer controlling his puppets. Watching a puppet show, you see only the smooth movements of the marionettes as they dance across the stage. You never see the hands above that direct every gesture of the puppets in front of you.

HGH is like the hand controlling the puppet, because HGH influences the functioning of the entire body. The puppeteer moves the marionette's arms, legs, and sometimes the mouth or eyes to create a certain facial expression, impacting all aspects of what we see. HGH is what energizes the organs and gives the body life and health. If there were no hand controlling the puppet's movement, the puppet would lie in an inanimate heap on the stage.

Of course, HGH is not the only element our bodies need to function well. For example, if the puppet is missing an arm or leg, the puppeteer can't make the marionette dance quite as smoothly. A puppet without a limb is like HGH without one of the other hormones or organs. When all the parts are there, the HGH puppeteer can influence and energize all of them. Overall, the puppeteer is still the variable that is the most influential in determining the final performance.

Several recent studies support the strong connection between HGH and the healthy functioning of the body. These studies indicate that adults with pituitary disease (HGH deficiency) have physical and psychological problems not found in healthy adults. These health problems remain despite therapy to raise the levels of adrenal, thyroid, and gonadal hormones. The problems of abnormal body composition, reduced strength and exercise capacity, reduced bone density, and higher cholesterol are conditions that are only addressed or corrected by optimal levels of growth hormone in the blood.[16]

Replacement therapy with corticosteroids and sex hormones has long been thought sufficient to treat a pituitary deficiency. But even with this treatment, patients with insufficient HGH still experienced a decrease in basal metabolism, a decline in renal

---

16 Powrie J, Weissberger A, Sonksen P. "Growth hormone replacement therapy for growth hormone-deficient adults." *Drugs* 49(5):656–663, 1995.

function, and a drop in blood volume and cardiac function.[17] These problems point directly to an HGH deficiency. It is only by replacing the missing HGH that we will see a significant improvement in an individual's overall health.

Research from around the world and results from the studies we've conducted at the Palm Springs Life Extension Institute confirm that HGH impacts all body systems and organs. HGH also helps keep all other hormones in line. By keeping these various components of the body running the same way it did when you were twenty years old, HGH does its job as the master hormone and the most powerful weapon we have in the war against aging.

ENDOCRINE SYSTEM

Every hormone has a specific job function and a particular message to carry to the cells throughout the body. For any hormone to be effective in its unique mission, it has to reach a receptor site on a cell, the place where the cell receives the message the hormone is carrying. HGH has been proven to increase the efficiency of the hormone receptor sites, allowing all the other hormones to work more effectively on all organs and in all parts of the body. The receptor site could be compared to a fax machine or phone. These instruments of communication are vital to the operation of most businesses and many homes. If the connections to these machines are not optimal, the messages come into the office incomplete or garbled. If the connections are repaired, the messages come through clearly and in their entirety. Just as this helps your business to function more efficiently, a good

17 Rosen T, Johannsson G, Johansson JO, Bengtsson, BA. "Consequences of growth hormone deficiency in adults and the benefits and risks of recombinant human growth hormone treatment." *Horm Res* 43:93–99, 1995.

connection between the hormones and the body's cells means improved communication and improved functioning.

HGH has the added power of stimulating some of the glands in the endocrine system to bring the production of other hormones up to optimal levels. In fact, this feature works both ways, demonstrating that all hormones work synergistically with each other. If DHEA, melatonin, and estrogen are all at their optimal levels, they can stimulate the pituitary gland to produce and secrete a greater amount of HGH, restoring it to its natural level. Also, since HGH reaches peak levels with nocturnal pulsatile secretion, sufficient sleep is vital to maintaining high HGH levels. If sleep patterns are disturbed, HGH may not be released and will never reach its peak. Melatonin, when in the body in sufficient amounts, restores normal sleep patterns, and in this way stimulates the natural, pulsatile release of HGH.

Growth hormone has a special and distinct role in the regulation of the thyroid hormone. Thyroid is responsible for energizing and providing fuel to the body. As it energizes all the body's functions, thyroid also regulates the body temperature, making sure you are not too hot or too cold. A thyroid deficiency shows up most prominently as a lack of energy and an inability to get warm. Studies have shown that patients with a thyroid deficiency also test positive for low levels of HGH. With HGH replacement, there is a corresponding increase in thyroid function and thyroid hormone metabolism. The relationship between growth hormone and thyroid hormone is also reciprocal. A balance of thyroid hormone stimulates HGH synthesis, secretion, and excretion.

IMMUNE SYSTEM

The endocrine system is most closely related to the immune system. In fact, their functions are so intertwined that the study of these two systems is often referred to collectively as immuno-endocrinology. Their main similarity is that they both help the body adjust quickly to the changing environment, fine-tuning the responses of each cell. For example, as part of the endocrine system, the thyroid hormone regulates body temperature. Without this adjustment, we would quickly freeze in chilly weather and overheat on a warm day. The adrenal gland responds to change by giving the body an extra boost of energy in an emergency. The immune system then does its part to help the body adjust by fighting off invaders.

Both systems work together to detect changes in the body and help each cell adapt. In order to do this, both the endocrine and immune systems must be in constant communication with each other. It only makes sense, then, that a healthy endocrine system, mastered by HGH, would be a strong influence in maintaining the health of the immune system.

Research has drawn a clear connection between HGH deficiency and the impairment of natural killer (NK) cell activity in both animals and humans. NK cells are the body's strongest defense against the spread of cancer. Researchers have suggested that HGH deficiency, resulting in fewer NK cells, may explain the increased incidence of tumors observed in the elderly.

But the connection between HGH and the immune system goes beyond NK cells and the ability to combat cancerous tumors. Research has found a clear relationship between HGH levels and the body's ability to fend off any disease. HGH deficiency has been shown to cause, or at least contribute to, immunodeficiency. Thus, HGH replacement is an effective therapy for improving the body's overall natural ability to defend itself against disease. Even if a person has enough NK cells and other immune system ammunition, there is experimental evidence to support that HGH therapy will enhance the activity of these, making them work even more quickly and efficiently to fight off infection and disease.

HGH therapy is, in fact, an immuno-stimulant because HGH helps manufacture new antibodies and T-cells. It also stimulates the output of white blood cells and increases production of red blood cells. A number of studies have demonstrated that HGH therapy helps patients fight off the infection from the skin allergy test used in the determination of biological age. HGH also reduces the incidence of infection occurring after surgery. Burn patients, for example, exhibit improved wound healing and have shortened hospital stays with HGH therapy.

The power of HGH in strengthening the immune system goes beyond even these dynamic benefits. HGH also has an amazing effect on one very small but very vital organ in our bodies. The thymus gland, located behind the breastbone, is a primary organ of the immune system. The thymus is important in the production of T-cells that defend the body against viruses and reject foreign tissue. But for some reason, this important organ begins shrinking at about age twelve, and by age sixty or seventy has all but disappeared. Similar to the declining hormone levels, the shrinking of the thymus has long been viewed as a normal part of life, and a physical phenomenon that we can do nothing about. However, researchers have linked the shrinking of the thymus with decreased manufacture of T-cells and the decreased immune function that we experience as we age, so restoring the thymus could help restore our immune system.

Dr. Keith Kelley, a researcher at the University of Illinois at Urbana-Champaign, noticed that just before the thymus begins to shrink, the blood serum levels of HGH are at their highest. This connection prompted his theory that replacing HGH levels could stimulate the regrowth of the thymus gland. He used old laboratory rats, whose thymus glands had shrunk in proportion to their age, and treated them with an HGH secretor. The shrunken gland amazingly regrew to the size of a thymus gland in a healthy young rat.[18]

The main agent in this regrowth may be insulin-like growth factor-1 (IGF-1) and not growth hormone itself. But HGH is what stimulates the production of the protein IGF-1. One of the many jobs of IGF-1 is to activate the thymus to produce T-cells. This connection led Dr. Ross Clark, an endocrinologist at Genentech Inc. in San Francisco, to believe that IGF-1 may also be the key to renewing the thymus. In animal studies, Dr. Clark found, "The thymus gland, which shrinks to one-half to one-quarter of its youthful size with age, can be made to bloom again with IGF-1."[19]

Replacing HGH to its optimal levels can be the first line of defense against disease. HGH stimulates and strengthens almost every facet of the immune system. If the immune system is healthy, the potential for illness is drastically reduced. Since the key to long life is avoiding illness, HGH therapy may be the answer to increasing the years of our lives and, more importantly, the *quality* of those years.

SKELETAL SUPPORT SYSTEM

The skeletal system is one part of our body that seems to be most taken for granted. We tend to ignore our bones until we notice a problem, and by then the problem is usually serious. Post-menopausal women taking estrogen supplements are probably the most appreciative of the importance of bone strength. For these women, the threat of

---

18 Kelley KW, Brief S, Westly HJ, et al. "GH3 pituitary adenoma cells can reverse thymic aging in rats." *Proc Natl Acad Sci USA* 83:5663–5667, 1986.

19 Brody J. "Restoring Ebbing Hormones May Slow Aging." *The New York Times* B5–6, 18 July 1995.

osteoporosis (porous bones) has suddenly become very real, and replacing estrogen can help counter this threat.

However, bone weakening threatens both men and women and is part of the illness called aging. A strong skeletal system is vital for many reasons. Strong bones give us greater mobility and are vital in protecting the body's precious organs. Imagine the damage you could cause to your spinal cord, heart, and lungs if your bones were not there to protect them just as stone walls protect the inhabitants of a medieval castle.

As with everything else in the body, skeletal strength is a matter of balancing two opposing forces. In this case, we're working with the osteoblasts, or bone growth stimulators, and the osteoclasts, which cause bone absorption. In the bodies of healthy children, these forces are balanced so that the osteoblasts have a greater edge over the osteoclasts. This is what allows bones to lengthen and children to grow taller during their physically formative years.

As old age approaches, this balance is thrown off, and osteoclasts become the stronger influence in our bodies. As a result, bone absorption accelerates, and the skeleton weakens. Bones affected by osteoporosis may break under the slightest pressure or during routine activities, greatly limiting physical ability. A common and dangerous type of injury resulting from osteoporosis is a hip fracture, which usually requires hospitalization and surgery and can be permanently debilitating. In fact, an average of 15 percent of osteoporosis sufferers die from simple hip fracture complications. Spinal or vertebral fractures may result in loss of height, severe back pain, and deformity.

Unfortunately, osteoporosis is not often diagnosed until such an injury occurs. Therefore it is important to pay attention to risk factors that may affect bone health, including diet, lifestyle, heredity, medication, certain chronic diseases, and, of course, hormone levels. If detected early, osteoporosis can be prevented and successfully treated. One of the most promising treatments is HGH replacement therapy.

HGH was originally named for its major role in helping children grow taller. It only makes sense, then, that human growth hormone has a direct connection to the forces controlling bone growth at any age. One symptom of HGH deficiency is a decrease in bone density. In fact, the decline in HGH is directly proportional to the loss of bone mass. Likewise, HGH replacement has been shown to cause a dramatic increase in bone strength in a relatively short time.

According to a German study, adults with HGH deficiency showed a reduction in bone mass of 51 percent in the lumbar spine and 73 percent in the forearm. This weakened structural state resulted in more bone fractures than normal.[20] An explanation for this weakening is the loss of bone mineral density also found in HGH-deficient adults. Growth hormone can return these minerals to the body, as evidenced by an increase in calcium levels after HGH replacement therapy.[21] This is because HGH helps the intestines absorb more calcium and phosphate from food. These minerals can then be used for strengthening our bones.[22]

---

20 Wuster C, Slenczka E, Ziegler R. "Increased prevalence of osteoporosis and arteriosclerosis in conventionally substituted anterior pituitary insufficiency: need for additional growth hormone substitution?" *Klin Wochenschr* 69(16):769–773, 1991.

21 Johansson AG, Burman P, Westermark K, et al. "The bone mineral density in acquired growth hormone deficiency correlates with circulating levels of insulin-like growth factor-1." *J Intern Med* 232:447–452, 1992.

22 Bouillon R. "Growth hormone and bone." *Horm Res* 36, Suppl 1:49–55, 1991.

Dr. Rudman's landmark 1990 study on HGH replacement in elderly men reported a 1.6 percent increase in lumbar vertebral bone density after only six months of treatment. These are the bones that protect our spinal cord, preserving the integrity of communication between the brain and the rest of the body. If these vertebral bones are strong, it improves the vital protection we need. If the rest of the bones in the skeletal system are strong, we will have the mobility and independence we need.[23]

For more information about osteoporosis, please contact:

National Osteoporosis Foundation
1232 22nd Street, N.W.
Washington, DC 20037-1292
Phone: (202) 223-2226
www.nof.org.

MUSCULAR SYSTEM

Working in conjunction with the skeletal system is the muscular system. They are often studied together as one system that is called the musculo-skeletal system. As I mentioned earlier, a strong skeletal system gives us greater mobility. Combine this with strong muscles, and your mobility and independence increase even more. Also, like the bones, muscles serve as protection for the organs.

Unfortunately, we lose this protection and mobility as our muscles weaken. It has been shown that muscle mass decreases

---

23 Brixen K, Kassem M, Nielsen HK, Loft AG, et al. "Short-term treatment with growth hormone stimulates osteoblastic and osteoclastic activity in osteopenic post-menopausal women: a dose response study." *J Bone Miner Res* 10(12):1865–1874, 1995.

Amato G, Izzo G, LaMontagna G, Bellastella A. "Low dose recombinant human growth hormone normalizes bone metabolism and cortical bone density and improves trabecular bone density in growth hormone deficient adults without causing adverse effects." *Clin Endocrinol (Oxf)* 45:27–32, 1996.

at a rate of one-half pound of muscle each year after age twenty. Exercise does help to increase strength, but many people find that even the healthiest exercise program is not enough for them to maintain the lifestyle they desire.

The key lies in increasing lean body (muscle) mass, or trying to replace that which has been lost over the years. Studies that evaluate HGH treatment in healthy adults have shown an impressive increase in fat-free mass (lean muscle) along with a corresponding decrease in fat mass. A study from the United Medical School in London concluded that this gain in lean body mass was due to an increase in HGH-stimulated protein synthesis. With this increase in muscle mass generally comes an increase in physical strength. Some studies have measured an increase in quadricep force after only four months of HGH replacement.[24]

Increased muscular strength, combined with the decrease in fat, has the helpful benefit of making everyday tasks easier. Climbing stairs and lifting objects become as easy as they were when you were in your twenties. But beyond helping with the daily tasks we encounter, strong muscles open the door to all kinds of activities that you may not have dared to do since you were a teenager. You may consider scuba diving or entering the dance contest you won thirty years ago.

This newfound agility is attributed to the skeletal muscles, which are responsible for your ease of movement and the strength of your limbs. Research shows that skeletal muscle constitutes 50 percent of lean body mass, so much of the overall body mass increase that hormone replacement patients experience is

---

24 Russell-Jones DL, Weissberger AH, Bowes SB, et al. "The effects of growth hormone on protein metabolism in adult growth hormone deficient patients." *Clin Endocrinol (Oxf)* 38(4):427–431, 1993.

undoubtedly due to the increase in skeletal muscle. In several studies, a cross-sectional computerized tomography scan of the thighs showed an increase of 5 percent to 8 percent in the muscle mass.[25]

A urine test that scans for a substance called creatinine can also serve as an indication of muscle mass. Creatinine is a white protein compound formed mostly in the muscles. The amount of creatinine that passes out of the body through the urine during a Twenty-four-hour period can give doctors a good indication of muscle mass. In Dr. Salomon's study, the amount of creatinine excretion rose after HGH treatment, indicating again that HGH stimulates an increase in muscle mass.

HGH's role in increasing muscle mass was discovered in an early study by D. B. Cheek and D. E. Hill. This study suggested that rather than increasing the size of the muscle cells in the body, growth hormone stimulates an overall increase in muscle mass by telling muscle cells to divide and therefore increase in number, strengthening the entire muscle.[26]

This increase in muscle cell mass is consistent with other studies by Bengt-Ake Bengtsson that showed an overall increase

---

25 Whitehead HM, Boreham C, McIlrath EM, et al. "Growth hormone treatment of adults with growth hormone deficiency: results of a 13-month placebo controlled cross-over study." *Clin Endocrinol* 36:45–52, 1992.

Jorgensen JO, Pedersen SA, Thuesen L, et al. "Beneficial effects of growth hormone treatment in GH-deficient adults." *Lancet* 1:1221–1225, 1989.

Cuneo RC, Salomon F, Wiles CM, et al. "Growth hormone treatment in growth hormone-deficient adults: I. Effects on muscle mass and strength." *J Appl Physiol* 70:688–694, 1991.

26 Cheek DB, Hill DE. "Effect of growth hormone on cell and somatic growth" in *Handbook of Physiology*. Greep RO, Astwood E, eds. Washington: American Physiological Society, 4(7):159–185, 1973.

in body cell mass of 6 percent after twelve months of growth hormone treatment.[27]

THE HEART

The most important muscle to strengthen is the heart. Conventionally, people endeavor to improve this muscle through aerobic exercise, but research shows that as the body ages, the heart is simply not able to withstand the stress of sustained exertion. Even in active people, the heart muscle weakens as hormone levels drop. Studies indicate that replacing these hormones, especially growth hormone, dramatically increases the health of the heart and the entire cardiovascular system. In fact, these studies give us some of the most exciting news about the incredible potential of growth hormone.[28]

As HGH replacement builds the muscles of the body, it also builds the muscles of the heart. A study from Italy indicates that in a patient with a weakened heart, the muscle mass of the left ventricle actually increased after only a short period of growth hormone therapy. Echocardiography shows the increase. This strengthened heart muscle improves the force of cardiac contractions or cardiac output. This means there is an increase in the volume of blood pushed through the heart each time it pumps. It is like giving a jack-in-the-box a new, tight spring. The jack-in-the-box jumps out quickly and with a lot of energy, but when the spring is worn out, it won't push the jack-in-the-box up

---

27 Rosen T, Johannsson G, Johansson JO, Bengtsson BA. "Consequences of growth hormone deficiency in adults and the benefits and risks of recombinant human growth hormone treatment." *Horm Res* 43:93–99, 1995.

28 Yang R, Bunting S, Gillett N, et al. "Effects of growth hormone in rats with postinfarction left ventricular dysfunction." *Cardiovasc Drugs Ther* 9(1):125–131, 1995.

as far or as fast. Strengthening the heart muscles helps the heart to work more efficiently and effectively, more like the tight spring. Because the muscle is working better, the patient also experiences an improvement in exercise performance.

A strong heart gives many of us new hope in the United States, where heart-related illnesses such as heart disease, heart attacks, and strokes are responsible for a majority of deaths. Rosen and Bengtsson of the University of Gothenberg recognized that patients who died of heart-related illnesses also showed a low level of growth hormone.[29]

Bengtsson's study of 333 patients with hypopituitarism showed a mortality rate almost double the expected number of deaths, and 60 percent of these deaths were attributed to cardiovascular disease. Many separate studies report an increase in the number of cardiovascular deaths among growth hormone-deficient adults, compared with other adults of similar age, sex, etc. with sufficient growth hormone in their body. This could be partially attributed to the hardening of arteries found in patients with hypopituitarism. These growth hormone-deficient adults have an increase in the number of atheromatous plaques in the arteries, or buildups caused by the fatty degeneration of the inner coat of the arteries. Most notably, these plaques were found in the vital femoral and carotid arteries that carry blood to the legs and head, respectively.[30]

Replacing the deficient growth hormone will both strengthen the heart muscles and clear the arteries of life threatening obstructions. A study performed by Dr. M. Volterrani of the

---

29 Rosen T, Bengtsson BA. "Premature mortality due to cardiovascular disease in hypopituitarism." *Lancet* 336:285–288, 1990.

30 Markussis V, Beshyah SA, Fisher C, et al. "Abnormal carotid compliance and distensibility in hypopituitarism." *Lancet* 340:1188–1192, 1992.

University of Brescia, Italy, studied twelve patients with chronic heart failure. He treated the patients, ages forty-nine to seventy-nine, with growth hormone and reported "a massive increase in cardiac output and an important drop in pulmonary resistance." Studies consistently show that growth hormone therapy increases left ventricular end-systolic dimension, stroke volume, and left ventricular myocardial mass. They confirm growth hormone's effectiveness in treating patients with serious heart problems such as severe cardiomyopathy.[31]

The benefits of growth hormone therapy to cardiac patients have been clearly demonstrated in a variety of settings and situations, with research evaluating the benefits in other settings every day. But the cardiovascular benefits of growth hormone therapy are not limited to individuals with cardiac damage. Studies have indicated that growth hormone plays a vital role in the maintenance of normal cardiac performance.

The consequences of growth hormone-deficient adults remaining untreated are striking. According to every study conducted in this population, untreated growth hormone-deficient adults suffer increased cardiovascular mortality, reduced exercise capacity, reduced muscle strength, defective stress secretions,

---

31 Capaldo B, Lembo G, Rendina V, et al. "Sympathetic deactivation by growth hormone treatment in patients with dilated cardiomyopathy." *Eur Heart J* 19(4):623–627, 1998.

Frustaci A, Perrone GA, Gentiloni N, et al. "Reversible dilated cardiomyopathy due to growth hormone deficiency." *Am J Clin Pathol* 97:503–511, 1992.

Lombardi G, Colao A, Cuocolo A, et al. "Cardiological aspects of growth hormone and insulin-like growth factor-1." *J Pediatr Endocrinol Metab* 10(6):553–560, 1997.

Osterzeil KJ, Markus U, Willenbrock R, et al. "Therapy of dilated cardiomyopathy with recombinant human growth hormone." *Z Kardiol* 86(10):803–811, 1997.

reduced energy expenditure, abnormal thyroid hormone metabolism, reduced myocardial function, and the clinical signs of premature atherosclerosis. They will also experience a change in body composition, with an increase in fat mass, a decrease in lean muscle mass, and a reduced bone mineral content. An individual's body weight and, more importantly, his or her cholesterol levels and body fat percentages are clearly serious risk factors for heart disease, as are most of the other conditions described above.

All of these deficiencies and abnormalities improve with growth hormone replacement, the only recognizable side effect being fluid retention. This has shown itself to be nearly universally transient and dose-dependent. In short, growth hormone deficiency has distinct cardiac consequences, all of which can be totally or partially alleviated by growth hormone replacement therapy.

LARGER CARDIOVASCULAR SYSTEM

Growth hormone also helps protect the body on another level: at each and every cell. Studies have shown that HGH protects cells from free radicals and other invaders. It is also believed that HGH can stimulate the reproduction of DNA in each cell. This cellular protection has proven very important in the case of a stroke. A heart attack or stroke is most frightening because of the damage it can do to the cells of the heart and brain, often causing cellular death. This damage can rob stroke victims of their mobility and their ability to speak, and leave them with a weakened heart and increased vulnerability to other heart problems. With sufficient HGH in the body, studies show that the cells of the heart and brain can be protected from death in the event of a stroke.

In the effort to keep our bodies healthy, our heart works very closely with our lungs, and growth hormone helps these essential organs as well. One of the tests to determine biological age involves measuring how much air a person can expel in one second. A 1991 study by Cuneo and colleagues studied the effects of growth hormone replacement on exercise performance. They indicated that growth hormone-deficient adults showed a maximum oxygen uptake that was reduced to about 80 percent of the healthy level. Maximum heart rate, with near maximum exertion, was only 90 percent of normal. After growth hormone treatment, both the maximum oxygen uptake and the maximum heart rate improved to healthy levels. This improved the individual's overall physical performance, especially with submaximal exertion, which is the effort category that includes most of our daily activities.[32]

Even sufferers of chronic obstructive pulmonary disease who have lost the ability to expand their lungs saw incredible improvements in forced vital capacity with growth hormone therapy. There is even some evidence that growth hormone can regrow lung tissue. The increase in lung capacity in turn increased the exercise abilities of patients. This is because, like a healthy heart, strong lungs are able to work more efficiently, getting oxygen to the cells more quickly and helping make the entire body healthier.

GASTROINTESTINAL SYSTEM

This system has not been studied as thoroughly as many of the others in relation to growth hormone influence. But a study done in 1995 measured the effect of the growth hormone glutamine, along with a modified diet, on patients with Severe Short Bowel Syndrome. This condition is characterized by poor intestinal absorption resulting in dehydration and malnutrition. The patients

32 Cuneo RC, Salomon F, Wiles CM, et al. "Growth hormone treatment in growth hormone-deficient adults: I. Effects on exercise performance." *J Appl Physiol* 70:695–700, 1991.

given the growth hormone regimen reported "an increase in the absorption of total calories, protein, carbohydrates, water, and sodium. Fat absorption did not change." This increased absorption helped the body make better use of the food it consumed. Getting the energy, minerals, and water out of the intestines and into the body cells means that they can now aid in building a healthier body. Growth hormone is a powerful agent in this process because it stimulates the intestinal cells to work better and carry out their specific duties as they would in a young, healthy body.[33]

KIDNEYS AND LIVER

Lung capacity was one of the tests listed in determining biological age. Another was the test of renal function, or how well the kidneys are working. This test is useful because kidney failure and the various ailments that go along with it become more and more common with age. The kidneys and the liver help rid the body of unwanted, unhealthy materials by filtering them out of the blood. The organ functions can be hampered by a history of drinking, injury to the organ, or the decline in cellular efficiency that comes with age. Studies as early as 1963 showed a definite decrease in the glomerular filtration rate and the renal (kidney) plasma flow in patients who were growth hormone-deficient. These patients' kidneys were not working as much or as efficiently as they do in a healthy body, and not all of the unwanted toxins were being cleaned out of the system.

Growth hormone has the power to rejuvenate the kidneys and the liver so that they function at an optimal level once more. The

---

33 Byrne TA, Morrissey TB, Nattakom TV, et al. "Growth hormone, glutamine, and a modified diet enhance nutrient absorption in patients with severe short bowel syndrome." *J Parenter Enteral Nutr* 19(4):296–302, 1995.

kidneys remove waste from the blood and help the body maintain the proper balance between salt and water. With age, the kidneys wear out, and we become more susceptible to kidney failure, a condition that can literally cause the body to poison itself. To treat kidney failure, patients must be put on dialysis, an expensive procedure by which the blood is pumped out of the body through a machine to filter out impurities. Most often, dialysis treatment takes place three times a week and continues for life, or until a donor kidney can be transplanted.

This is a long, painful, and life-threatening process that could be avoided, or at least delayed, by the use of growth hormone. Studies with patients who have suffered renal injuries show that replacing HGH increases glomerular filtration, helping the kidneys to filter out more of the body's poison. A study from the Harbor-UCLA Medical Center revealed that growth hormone treatment normalized glomerular function in growth hormone-deficient rats. The treatment also increased kidney weight. Growth hormone also has the ability to fight off the toxins directly, decreasing the amount of nitrogenous waste in the blood that the kidneys have to process. This reduces the overall stress on the kidneys, thereby prolonging their useful life.[34]

The catabolism and consequent malnutrition that slows healing in burn, trauma, and surgical patients can be life-threatening for people with acute or end-stage kidney disease. When body wasting and malnutrition are added to these already dire health problems, the patient's very survival is threatened. In

34 Hirschberg R. "Effects of growth hormone and IGF-1 on glomerular ultra filtration in growth hormone-deficient rats." *Regul Pept* 48(1–2):241–250, 1993.

O'Shea M, Miller SB, Finkel K, Hammerman MR. "Roles of growth hormone and growth factors in the pathogenesis and treatment of kidney disease." *Curr Opin Nephrol Hypertens* 2(1):67–72, 1993.

several published studies involving kidney failure patients, human growth hormone's anticatabolic assistance was a lifesaver.

In one such study by Tokyo Women's Medical College in Japan, HGH was administered to malnourished, end-stage renal disease (ESRD) patients to establish the therapeutic effect on the patients' nutritional states. According to the study, patients in the group receiving HGH showed a significantly higher improvement in their nutritional states than the control group. This study was good news for ESRD patients who know that good nutrition has always translated into improved survival rates.[35]

Growth hormone replacement can similarly aid in the functioning of the liver. The liver is a large organ, weighing about three pounds. It is the chemical center of the body and performs two major functions. The first is the conversion of sugar into lipids and carbohydrates that are then stored for the body to use between meals. This function is absolutely vital to brain performance and the workings of the central nervous system, since they are both fueled only by the sugar process in the liver. Similar to the kidneys, the liver also works as a filter, cleaning toxic substances out of the blood. The liver can be weakened through infection, alcohol consumption, or injury, causing liver disease. This then stresses the kidneys by leaving them to do the entire job of ridding the body of toxins.

Because liver disease, or cirrhosis, is a condition resulting from the collective damage in many individual cells of the liver, growth hormone can help repair these cells. This has been shown in many studies, including a recent one reported by Sheffield University in

---

35 Shinobe M, Sanaka T, Nihei H, Sugino N. "IGF-1/IGFBP-1 as an index for discrimination between responder and nonresponder to recombinant human growth hormone in malnourished uremic patients on hemodialysis." *Nephron* 77(1):29–36, 1997.

England, where researchers reported that "patients with end-stage liver failure respond to supraphysiological doses of HGH."[36]

However, there is a point of diminishing return, at which the damage has gone too far and spread for so long that growth hormone's restorative powers may not have as great an influence. In spite of this, the anabolic properties of growth hormone positively affect protein metabolism, suggesting that HGH therapy could be used to treat those with chronic liver disease. Growth hormone improves other liver functions because it stimulates the LDL (bad) cholesterol receptor sites in the liver. These receptor sites then are able to pull more of the unwanted cholesterol out of the blood, and eventually out of the body. This lowers the body's overall LDL cholesterol level.

SKIN AND HAIR

When you first see an elderly person, how do you know they are old? Often, it is the person's appearance that first suggests age. You notice wrinkles and gray hair long before you are aware of any diseases, memory loss, or lack of energy.

Because of this, many people are as concerned about their physical appearance as they are about interior health, or more so. As evidence of this universal desire to look twenty years old, wrinkle creams, hair coloring, youth formulas, and costly plastic surgeries are big business. People are eager to plunk down money for anything that will guarantee youth in a bottle. Some of these products use natural ingredients that work to replace some of what the body has lost. Often these formulas help, but they are not sufficient to reverse the damage that has already been done.

---

36 Shen XY, Holt RI, Miell JP, et al. "Cirrhotic liver expresses low levels of the full-length and truncated growth hormone receptors." *J Clin Endocrinol Metab* 83(7):2532–2538,1998.

So the quest for youth leads a large part of the aging population to options like plastic and laser surgery.

But none of these solutions is adequate. Instead, we must first discover what causes the skin and hair to show signs of aging, and then stop the forces behind the damage. Wrinkles, for example, appear as the skin thins, dries, and loses its elasticity. The outer layer of skin on our bodies, the epidermis, and the cells in this layer have the unique ability to divide and replicate an infinite number of times. But underneath the epidermis is a layer called the dermis, where each cell is programmed to divide only a certain number of times. When the cell stops dividing, it dies. The older we get, the fewer healthy live cells we have in the dermis. This is what causes the skin to thin, lose its elasticity, and wrinkle.

Though technology is not quite to the point where we can prevent the death of the dermis cells, we can use growth hormone to repair much of the damage. As it does in virtually every part of the body, growth hormone stimulates new cell growth and strengthens and protects the existing cells, making the old cells act like new. In Dr. Rudman's study, he noticed that growth hormone therapy caused an increase in both dermal and epidermal thickness. Replacing growth hormone improves the collagen synthesis in the body. Collagen is a protein contained in the connective tissue of the body, somewhat like a glue that holds things together. Collagen synthesis declines with age, causing the skin to sag. Increase that synthesis, and the skin is lifted back into its proper place and held there.

We have shown how growth hormone stimulates muscle growth. HGH does the same for the muscles just underneath the skin, especially the facial muscles. Strengthening the facial muscles helps to tighten the skin that covers them, eliminating fine lines and wrinkles. Growth hormone also decreases the amount of fat in the body, including the deposits underneath the skin. Reducing this fat is another way to help the skin regain its youthful appearance.

With growth hormone, you are really performing a form of *medical* cosmetic plastic surgery. But it is completely natural. Growth hormone patients report an almost immediate improvement in the thickness of their skin, with fewer fine lines and wrinkles, and improved elasticity. The overall result is a younger face and smoother, firmer skin on the entire body.

Since hair loss and graying hair are also almost exclusively tied to aging, growth hormone can often affect these as positively as it does the skin. In early studies at the Palm Springs Life Extension Institute, 38 percent of our patients reported an overall improvement in hair thickness and texture. In some cases, natural hair color returned, and a few people even experienced hair regrowth.

Growth hormone has the power not only to make you feel better by fixing what has deteriorated on the inside of the body, but it can also make you look better by giving your outside a new finish. Looking at someone who has been on growth hormone therapy, even the most discerning eye would have trouble determining the individual's true chronological age.

WOUND HEALING AND SURGICAL RECOVERY

Several studies have shown that growth hormone is a significant positive influence in helping the body heal. In fact, growth hormone has been used in hospitals to help surgical patients recover from their wounds faster. The first clinical studies describing the administration of human growth hormone to postoperative and post-traumatic patients date back to the early 1960s. By 1990, an increasing number of papers had reported the positive influence of HGH on wound healing, especially skin grafts, septic conditions, burns, and traumatic injuries. An increased understanding of the body's response to trauma has again made human growth hormone the topic of several new studies in these areas.

Physicians are now aware that infection, trauma, surgery, and most major illnesses all cause a kind of body wasting, a type of muscle and weight loss called protein catabolism. This condition can seriously slow the body's ability to heal. In a recent report, physicians described using human growth hormone to successfully treat catabolism in patients undergoing abdominal surgery.[37]

Other recent animal studies with growth hormone reported incidences of actual regeneration of intestinal tract length and accelerated recovery after surgery that removed large amounts of the intestinal tract. This holds out hope that HGH may assist in better recovery in patients with a wide array of devastatingly invasive and debilitating gastrointestinal surgeries.[38]

A similar study from Denmark tested the effects of growth hormone treatment on rats with experimental colitis. The rats that received the growth hormone showed overall less macroscopic and microscopic damage, and they were able to regain their initial body weight after only seven days of treatment. In comparison, the control group remained 11 percent below their initial body weight.[39]

---

37 Bjarnason R, Wickelgren R, Hermansson M, et al. "Growth hormone treatment prevents the decrease in insulin-like growth factor-1 gene expression in patients undergoing abdominal surgery." *J Clin Endocrinol Metab* 83(5):1566–1572, 1998.

38 Iannoli P, Miller JH, Ryan CK, et al. "Epidermal growth factor and human growth hormone accelerate adaptation after massive enterectomy in an additive, nutrient-dependent, and site-specific fashion." *Surgery* 122(4):721–728, 1997.

39 Christensen H, Flyvbjerg A, Orskov H, Laurberg S. "Effect of growth hormone on the inflammatory activity of experimental colitis in rats." *Scand J Gastronenterol* 28(6):503–511, 1993.

Recovery involves much more than regaining lost weight. Since growth hormone stimulates body cell division, it makes sense that everything from paper cuts and abrasions to broken bones and torn internal tissue would heal faster with sufficient growth hormone in the system to stimulate it. Growth hormone also helps to strengthen each individual cell, so that the injury heals healthily, and often with less scarring. This explains the use of growth hormone to treat recovering burn victims.

The muscle-building effects of growth hormone are also extremely beneficial in injury situations. Often, an injury victim cannot use the injured muscle throughout the duration of the healing process, resulting in a weak, atrophied muscle that takes a great deal of physical therapy to strengthen again. Growth hormone cuts down on this recovery time by building and strengthening the muscle, even when the patient can't move it.

EYESIGHT

The effect of growth hormone on vision has been documented at the Palm Springs Life Extension Institute. Many people experience problems with their vision as they age. We have received increasing reports of individuals on growth hormone who one day realize they no longer need their reading glasses. This may be the result of improvement in the strength of the ciliary muscles that control the lens, or reversal of macular degeneration.

Macular degeneration is the leading cause of blindness for those fifty-five and older. Although it's more common in people over sixty, it is possible to develop symptoms in your forties or fifties. There are two types of macular degeneration, but 70 percent to 90 percent of the cases are caused by aging and thinning of the tissues of the macula. A healthy macula allows us to see fine detail and is necessary for driving, reading, recognizing faces, and doing close work, such as sewing.

Research is currently underway investigating the effectiveness of human growth hormone, antioxidants, and a low-fat diet as ways of preventing macular degeneration. The HGH approach makes a lot of sense because of its ability to regenerate and restore thickness and elasticity to aging tissues.

GROWTH HORMONE AND SEX

One of the universal reports of patients who are on growth hormone therapy is that their sex lives drastically improved. Growth hormone has the ability to stimulate the other hormones, including the sex hormones, resulting in a greatly enhanced libido. Suddenly, people who seemed to have lost their appetite for sex now enjoy as much sexual energy as a person one-third their age.

Sexual disinclination and dysfunction is another of those age-related changes that many people accept as normal and inevitable. The normality of it, however, does not eliminate the frustration people feel as they go through it themselves. A person who was once sexually vivacious finds that he or she no longer has the energy for sex—and worse, the desire has also diminished. Some men find they can no longer get an erection, and women have difficulty lubricating. All of these changes can be traced back to declining hormone levels.

In a study of 172 men receiving growth hormone at the Palm Springs Life Extension Institute, three quarters of the group reported a dramatic increase in libido, and more than half said they were able to maintain an erection for a longer period of time. Women on replacement therapy have also reported a dramatic increase in sexual desire and energy, accompanied by more intense, even multiple, orgasms. The increased energy is a direct result of growth hormone strengthening the various body systems and energizing the thyroid hormone. The maximized pleasure could be caused by growth hormone energizing the nervous system. An improved desire can be attributed to growth hormone's influence on sex hormones.

As growth hormone can reverse shrinkage in organs like the heart and thymus, it apparently has the same effect on sexual organs. Results from many of our patients indicate that in restoring hormone levels to those of a twenty-year-old, the man's penis and the woman's clitoris will return to their original size. A 1996 study from the Mayo Clinic showed that growth hormone therapy alone could restore normal phallic size in HGH-deficient men.[40]

Growth hormone is able to rejuvenate sexual function on several levels. In one study from Japan's Hamamatsu University School of Medicine, Japanese urologists reported that men with sexual problems often have low testosterone and growth hormone levels, and that HGH plays an important role in restoring normal sexual function in a variety of sexual and reproductive difficulties. This research supports our patients' claims about human growth hormone revitalizing their sex lives.[41]

Another study indicated that HGH treatment increased sperm motility significantly in men who were previously considered infertile.[42]

We've already talked about the positive effects that growth hormone treatment has on body composition, skin, and hair. And

40 Levy JB, Husmann DA. "Micropenis secondary to growth hormone deficiency: does treatment with growth hormone alone result in adequate penile growth?" *J Urol* 156(1):214–216, 1996.

41 Fujita K, Terada H, Ling LZ. "Male sexual insufficiency." *Nippon Rinsho* 55(11):2908–2913, 1997.

42 Ovesen P, Jorgensen JO, Ingerslev J, et al. "Growth hormone treatment of subfertile males." *Fertil Steril* 66(2):292–298, 1996.

an improved physical appearance, from stronger muscles to fewer wrinkles, can also improve our sexual confidence. With adequate levels of human growth hormone, all of the separate systems in the body work together to keep individuals at their physical, and therefore sexual, best.

With proper hormone treatment, patients report that sex is better now than when they were in their twenties. This treatment does come with a friendly word of caution, however. It is most satisfactory when both partners are taking part in the hormone replacement program. Only slightly less frustrating than the loss of libido altogether is the discovery that the desires and responses of your spouse or significant other do not measure up to your own. When both of you are on a growth hormone replacement program, you can share the great benefits of sexual rejuvenation.

THE BRAIN

Many of the benefits of growth hormone therapy that we have already described also apply to the brain and the central nervous system. HGH has the ability to protect and strengthen each cell in the body, including the brain cells, based on studies with stroke victims. It is also possible that a growth hormone deficiency may be partly to blame for the brain shrinkage that occurs as we age. Since growth hormone has proven abilities to increase nerve growth factors, the probability exists that by replacing human growth hormone to optimal levels, we could also rebuild precious brain cells.

Growth hormone does have many proven brain-enhancing functions. For example, growth hormone can increase the concentration of neurotransmitters in the brain. The greater the concentration of neurotransmitters, the quicker the transfer of information in the brain, and the quicker the response time.

Because of the increased concentration of neurotransmitters, patients reported greater overall mental acuity. But even more common were the reports of improved memory, which can also be attributed to a greater neurotransmitter concentration. Many of us have said or have heard people say, “I can’t remember. I must be getting old.” Loss of memory has long been linked to aging, and now researchers have found a direct link between memory skills and the amount of growth hormone in the body.

FEELING WELL

This news gives many of us great hope, since for much of the aging population, the fear of losing mental abilities can be even more frightening than the loss of physical skills. Growth hormone has the ability to protect both the mind and the body from the ravages of time. Along with protecting the brain and returning some mental abilities, growth hormone also seems to give people back an overall feeling of youth and a sense of well-being. The old saying, “You’re only as old as you feel,” suddenly takes on new meaning, as growth hormone recipients report that they are more energetic and feel as if they can do anything in the world.

As a whole, adults who are growth hormone-deficient do not feel this enthusiasm for life. In fact, surveys filled out by the patients indicate that they see themselves as having many more physical and mental problems than the average person. They complain of low energy levels, emotional instability, and social isolation. The fatigue, inability to concentrate, and memory difficulties can also impair an individual’s work skills, affecting not only career and social status, but also self image. A study by McGauley, Cuneo, and Salomon reported that more than a third of these growth hormone-deficient patients scored psychologically in a range that would normally warrant professional psychiatric treatment. A follow-up study indicated that some patients saw an increase in energy levels after only one week on growth hormone therapy; after six months, patient questionnaires confirmed an overall improvement in psychological well-being.[43]

From self-assessment questionnaires given to patients at the Palm Springs Life Extension Institute, we noted a significant improvement in mood and memory. Respondents indicated that they felt they had regained an energy they hadn't felt since their twenties, that they felt more emotionally stable, and had a greatly improved attitude toward life. They also noted that memory skills were significantly enhanced.

These observations suggest that growth hormone might also work as an antidepressant in the brain. In a study of major depressive illness, Fiasche and colleagues from Argentina determined that a low level of growth hormone corresponded with neurotransmitter impairment, resulting in the illness. Rejuvenating growth hormone levels to their optimal level may then stimulate the neurotransmitters and conquer major depressive illness.[44]

The improved psychological condition could also be attributed, at least in part, to the dramatic physical improvements that patients can see and feel. They lose fat and gain muscle, have more energy and better mental speed, meaning that they can do more with their lives. This is bound to make them feel better about themselves and the world as a whole.

---

43 McGauley GA, Cuneo RC, Salomon F, et al. "Psychological well-being before and after growth hormone treatment in adults with growth hormone deficiency." *Horm Res* 33 Suppl 4:52–54, 1990.

44 Fiasche R, Fideleff HL, Moisezowicz J, Frieder P, Pagano SM, Holland M. "Growth hormone neurosecretory dysfunction in major depressive illness." *Psychoneuroendocrinology* 20(7):727–733, 1995.

CHAPTER 8

HGH Adjunct Therapy in Disease

OBESITY, THE PLAGUE OF THE TWENTIETH CENTURY

Watch any thirty minutes of daytime television, from the early morning news to the talk shows to the soaps, and you will be hit with a barrage of advertising aimed at helping you lose those unwanted pounds. There are specific diet and counseling programs that charge a monthly, weekly, or by-the-pound fee. There are low-calorie shakes that are supposed to fill you up like a regular meal. And there are any number of pills that promise to make you lose the desire to eat unhealthy snacks. This bombardment of happy, energetic, and (most importantly) thin people that litters the airwaves and newsstands is aimed at the approximately fifty-eight million Americans (an alarming third of the population) who are overweight or obese.

Are you part of the growing population who resolves each January 1 to lose weight? A simple way to determine your fat fitness is the waist-to-hip ratio test. To find this ratio, measure your waist (at the smallest area below your rib cage and above your navel) and your hips (at the widest point). Divide waist measurement by hip measurement to get your waist-to-hip ratio. A ratio of 1.0 or more is in the danger zone.

Guidelines from the National Institutes of Health state that if the body mass index is more than twenty-five, you are also considered overweight. Thirty or higher is considered obese.

Body mass index can be determined as follows:

Calculate your BMI by dividing weight in pounds by height in inches squared, and then multiplying by a conversion factor of 703.

$$\frac{(703 \text{ x Body Weight, in Pounds})}{(\text{Height, in Inches})^2}$$

For Example: Weight = 180 lbs, Height = 5'8"

Calculation: $200 \div (65)^2 \text{ x } 703 = 27.4$

Being overweight is usually seen as a cosmetic or appearance problem. After all, that's what advertising focuses on. But in reality, being overweight (having a hip-to-waist ratio of more than 1.0) dangerously increases the risk of heart disease and stroke, even in the absence of other risk factors (genetic tendencies, for example). People who are overweight are also more likely to get diabetes and have trouble with arthritis. So not only would weight loss improve your physical appearance, but shedding those pounds could also save your life. No wonder dieting is such a big business.

But for many people, even with the aid of professional counselors, dieting doesn't solve the problem. They may temporarily lose weight, but they almost always gain it back. As we age, it becomes more and more difficult to fit into our old clothes, and parts of our bodies start to bulge and hang out in ways we would never have imagined. And no matter how we try, no matter how well we eat or how much we exercise, those extra pounds and that baggage around the middle stays with us. Many people say this is a normal part of aging that we just have to get used to.

But we don't. There is a very simple way to fight the fat war without the ammunition of appetite-control drugs, skimpy shakes, or weight loss centers. First, we have to understand why we gain weight. As with everything else in our bodies, weight gain is a matter of imbalance. Obesity may be caused by excess calorie intake, or a decrease in metabolism or hormone levels, resulting in fat storage. In short, we gain fat because the body's metabolic forces are no longer balanced. The body can no longer work efficiently enough to use up all the fat that it receives.

And one of the hormones that controls metabolism is none other than the amazing human growth hormone.

Studies show a direct correlation between obesity and low levels of HGH. A 1996 study from the Netherlands showed that, compared to people of the same age with healthy levels of growth hormone, HGH-deficient adults had 75 percent greater skinfold measurements and 84 percent more intra-abdominal fat. Likewise, every study involving HGH replacement, from Dr. Rudman to more recent studies, indicates that a decrease in the percentage of body fat is dramatic and almost immediate.

In our studies, we have found that obese patients can lose as much as 10 percent to 12 percent of their body fat, depending on their overall body composition, every six months they are on an HGH replacement therapy program. A person who is excessively overweight (for example, five feet four inches tall and weighing two hundred pounds) can lose twenty-four pounds of fat every six months. The percentages are lower for those who are overweight but not obese. Another study from St. Thomas Hospital in London showed a reduction in fat mass of 18 percent over a period of six months, with the most drastic improvement taking place during the first month of therapy. The Dutch study showed that the sum of skinfold measurements decreased by 27 percent, and abdominal fat was reduced an amazing 47 percent after HGH treatment.[45]

Normally, people who diet and lose weight this quickly will almost as quickly gain it back, usually with the addition of extra pounds. The difference with HGH is that it works with your body, not just to get rid of the fat, but to change the message your body receives on how specifically to use the fat. HGH binds with the fat in the body, triggering its breakdown and making it available for use. It breaks down triglycerides into glycerol and free fatty acids. This fat no longer needs to be stored, since it can now be used to fuel the body rather than slow it down.

The deposits of fat that accumulate around so many aging midsections are probably the most dangerous stores of fat in the body. Studies show that people who are HGH-deficient have an average of 7 percent excess fat, and the majority of that fat gathers around the abdomen. People who carry excess weight around the waist (abdominal fat) have a greater risk of heart disease and cancer than those who are pear-shaped and carry their weight around the hips. Bengt-Ake Bengtsson and his colleagues discovered that HGH not only reduces the overall body fat, but specifically targets abdominal fat, decreasing it by as much as 30 percent in six months. In comparison, other areas of the body lost 13 percent

45 de Boer H, Blok GJ, Voerman B, et al. "Changes in subcutaneous and visceral fat mass during growth hormone replacement therapy in adult men." *Int J Obes Relat Metab Disord* 20(6):580–587, 1996.

of their body fat. This thinning in the middle restores the normal body composition that we see in young, healthy individuals.[46]

Another factor in the loss of body fat may be the body's basal metabolic rate. Often we hear people say that they could lose weight if only they had a higher metabolism. This magical, mysterious word refers to the rate at which heat is given off by a body at rest. In other words, this is how fast and effectively the body works without needing to be stimulated with exercise. The higher your basal metabolic rate, the better your body is using the fuel it receives. In fact, many people with a high metabolism (particularly teenagers and young adults) can eat large quantities of food and not gain weight. For many of them, that amount of food is necessary to fuel the everyday functioning of the body. HGH-deficient adults characteristically have a very low basal metabolic rate. But studies indicate an increase in basal metabolic rate of 22 percent after one month of HGH treatment, with the rate staying at 16 percent above pre-treatment levels after six months of therapy.

Incredibly, the characteristics of HGH allow not only for fat loss, but also for muscle gain. The goal is to decrease the body fat percentage and increase the amount of lean muscle mass in the body. Most weight loss programs and diets focus on what the scale says, resulting in as much as or more of a loss of muscle mass as of body fat. But because HGH is striving to get the entire body back into balance and is not just fighting the fat, patients do not experience a decrease in muscle mass as they lose body fat. In fact, they put on muscle mass at the rate of 8 percent to 10 percent every six months.

More recent research continues to support HGH's reputation as a builder of better bodies. In a study published in May 1998,

---

46 Bengtsson BA, Eden S, Lonn L, et al. "Treatment of adults with growth hormone (GH) deficiency with recombinant human growth hormone." *J Clin Endocrinol Metab* 76:309–317, 1993.

HGH once again showed its ability to restore youthful, lean bodies while increasing muscle strength. For this research, post-menopausal women participated in a randomized double-blind study to determine the effects of growth hormone when added to a diet and exercise program. Weight loss, decreased fat, and increased muscle strength were consistently most significant in the group taking growth hormone.[47]

But let's remember that thyroid hormone and epinephrine (adrenal) hormone also control the metabolism and the percentage of body fat. These hormones need to be balanced before the HGH replacement will work. In fact, the Palm Springs Life Extension Institute is the first in the world to advocate measuring epinephrine deficiencies as the cause of obesity. And the weight loss and muscle building that follow HGH therapy are important for more than just the sake of a smaller waist. When the body returns to a healthy, muscular weight, the body's long-term cardiovascular strength is increased, and the chance of heart disease is significantly decreased.[48]

REDUCING CHOLESTEROL LEVELS

Combined with this dramatic loss of body fat is the reduction in LDL (bad) cholesterol levels in the body. High levels of this cholesterol are life threatening and increase your chances of heart disease, fat buildup in the arteries, and stroke. Many Americans are currently on

---

47 Thompson JL, Butterfield GE, Gylfadottir UK, et al. "Effects of human growth hormone, insulin-like growth factor-1, and diet and exercise on body composition of obese post-menopausal women." *J Clin Endocrinol Metab* 83(5):1477–1484, 1998.

48 Binnerts A, Swart GR, Wilson JH, et al. "The effect of growth hormone administration in growth hormone deficient adults on bone protein, carbohydrate and lipid homeostasis, as well as on body composition." *Clin Endocrinol (Oxf)* 37:79–87, 1992.

restrictive diets and medication to help control their blood cholesterol levels. But HGH battles this killer by stimulating the LDL cholesterol receptor sites in the liver. These receptor sites are then able to filter the blood better and take the unwanted cholesterol out of the body entirely.[49] In looking at approximately one hundred fifty patients from the Palm Springs Life Extension Institute, the mean and the median showed a twenty-point drop on the cholesterol scale. Also, at the 50th percentile range, triglycerides decreased significantly, with patients experiencing a thirty- to forty-point drop

OSTEOARTHRITIS AND FIBROMYALGIA

Along with osteoporosis, age-related arthritis (osteoarthritis) is one of the most life-quality reducing symptoms many people face as they age. This debilitating condition is characterized by pain and reduction in movement, accompanied by an inability to perform simple activities and everyday duties. Osteoarthritis is a condition primarily in the weight-bearing joints, in which the cartilage that covers the ends of bones in the joint deteriorates, causing pain and loss of movement as bone begins to rub against bone.

Research has established a definite connection between low levels of HGH and the incidence of osteoarthritis. High levels of HGH encourage cartilage growth, so a hormone deficiency probably causes cartilage loss. Since HGH encourages cartilage growth, it's an ideal treatment for osteoarthritis. HGH has the added power of being able to reverse the damage already caused by cartilage loss. After all, you didn't have osteoarthritis when you were twenty.

---

49 Rudling M, Norstedt F, Olivecrona H, et al. "Importance of growth hormone for the induction of hepatic low density lipoprotein receptors." *Proc Nat Acad Sci USA* 89:6983–6987, 1992.

Snyder DK, Underwood LE, Clemmons DR. "Persistent lipolytic effect of exogenous growth hormone during caloric restriction." *Am J Med* 98(2):129–134, 1995.

Another condition that is becoming more and more common is fibromyalgia. In the case of fibromyalgia, widespread pain affects the muscles and attachments to the bone, again limiting the movement and abilities of sufferers. As with osteoarthritis, fibromyalgia patients show significantly lower than normal levels of growth hormone, and HGH therapy has proven to be an effective treatment.

HGH also battles rheumatoid arthritis by boosting the immune system. As we discussed in relation to the immune system, IGF-1 stimulates the production of T-cells in the thymus gland. These defenders fight off bacteria and cancer. This arthritis is, in fact, a self-attack autoimmune disease in which there is a breakdown in the immune system's ability to recognize its own cells—in this case, the membrane that lines the joint surfaces.

Rheumatoid arthritis attacks symmetrical joints, such as the fingers, wrists, feet, and knees, and can also attack areas outside of the joints including kidneys, eyes, heart, and lungs. This characteristic of rheumatoid arthritis means that the disease not only threatens the quality of life, but can also threaten life itself. In fact, studies show a reduced life expectancy of three to seven years for rheumatoid arthritis sufferers.

Returning your HGH levels to those of a twenty-year-old could strengthen the immune system and add those years and more back on to your life.

SLEEP: STOP COUNTING SHEEP

A common symptom of HGH deficiency is sleep disorder, including decreased REM sleep, increased total sleep time, and severe daytime drowsiness. It is not thoroughly understood exactly how HGH affects our sleep patterns, but it has been proven that HGH treatment increases the length of the REM stage of sleep. Doctors have determined that REM sleep is the most physically beneficial. But amazingly, although HGH treatment increased the REM sleep time by twenty-seven minutes, the total sleep time needed by patients was decreased. With this came a significantly improved sense of well-being, and an increase in daytime energy.[50]

DIABETES: THE SUGAR IMBALANCE

Along with loss of energy, strength, and sexual appetite, and an increase in the risk of heart disease, aging brings with it a greater chance of developing diabetes.

One of the earliest observed side effects of HGH replacement was its effect on insulin and blood sugar levels. Many HGH therapy patients do experience some initial increase in insulin and blood sugar levels in glucose tolerance tests. But these changes in blood sugar levels are temporary, lasting anywhere from three to six months. In fact, by the end of twelve months, many patients on hormone replacement therapy completely normalize their insulin resistance.[51]

And in the long run, the diabetic patient can benefit from HGH therapy. HGH increases insulin receptor sensitivity, making less

---

50 Astrom C, Lindholm J. "Growth hormone-deficient young adults have decreased deep sleep." *Neuroendocrinology* 51:82–84, 1990.

Astrom C, Christensen L, Gjerris F, Trojaborg W. "Sleep in acromegaly before and after treatment with adenectomy." *Neuroendocrinology* 53:328–331, 1992.

Astrom C, Pedersen SA, Lindholm J. "The influence of growth hormone on sleep in adults with growth hormone deficiency." *Clin Endocrinol* 33:495–500, 1990.

Mendelson WB, Slater S, Gold P, Gillin JC. "The effect of growth hormone administration on human sleep: a dose-response study." *Biol Psychiatry* 15:613–616, 1980.

51 Hwu CM, Kwok CF, Lai TY, et al. "Growth hormone (GH) replacement reduces total body fat and normalizes insulin sensitivity in GH-deficient adults: a report of one-year clinical experience." *J Clin Endocrinol Metab* 82(10):3285–3292, 1997.

insulin necessary to carry out the transfer of glucose from our blood into our cells. The additional benefit to the diabetic is HGH's alteration of body composition. We have already shown that HGH increases muscle mass and reduces body fat. When diabetics experience these changes, their insulin requirements are lowered even more. Indeed, with insulin sensitivity related to total fat, it is important to note that HGH treatment leads to a reduction in central fat, percent fat, total fat, and in the waist-to-hip ratio. Also, HGH treatment significantly increases HDL (good) cholesterol levels, while contributing to a minor overall decrease in cholesterol levels.

Wound healing is also a more profound problem for diabetics than for the general population, and growth hormone can help there as well. In several recently published studies, HGH has been documented to actively encourage healing in diabetics.[52]

Of course, extra care should be given to diabetic patients who are undergoing HGH treatment, and their conditions must be monitored closely, since they can develop hypoglycemia after four to six months of HGH treatment if their insulin or anti-diabetic medication is not reduced. But all indications are that the diabetic patient has everything to gain from HGH replacement therapy.

MALNUTRITION IN AGING

One aspect of aging that we have not discussed is malnutrition. One of the sad realities of the aging population is that they very often suffer from malnutrition, which is too often unrecognized and even more often inadequately treated. Malnutrition affects the daily activities and abilities of virtually every aging individual, and complicates the other difficulties of aging.

---

52 Massey KA, Blakeslee C, Pitkow HS. "Possible therapeutic effects of growth hormone on wound healing in the diabetic patient." *J Am Podiatr Assoc* 88(1):25–29, 1998.

Reduced secretion of HGH has been recognized as being a direct cause of malnutrition. While weight loss is more typical of well-nourished patients, hormone replacement therapy has been shown to cause both weight and muscle gain in malnourished patients, with virtually no side effects. In one study, body weight increased by more than five pounds. Many researchers believe that even with adequate nutritional intake, underweight elderly patients could greatly benefit from low-dose HGH replacement, which helps the body more efficiently absorb all the nutrients in the food that is consumed. One contributing factor is the increased intestinal absorption that accompanies HGH replacement. If the intestines are doing their job right, the vitamins, minerals, and carbohydrates from the food we eat will get into the body and be used to nourish each cell.

AIDS: NEW HOPE

Many of the symptoms of aging are also characteristics of acquired immune deficiency syndrome (AIDS). Watching someone suffer with AIDS is like watching someone age very rapidly. The AIDS sufferer quickly grows weak, the muscles, bones, and skin all deteriorate, and the body can no longer fight off diseases. We have proven that HGH can help counter these problems in the aging individual, and while HGH therapy may not be a cure for AIDS, it can help alleviate some of its symptoms.

Studies in 1990 by Jospe and Laue both noted that classic HGH deficiency existed in several HIV-positive children. These studies, and several others, indicate that HGH secretion and activity in HIV-positive individuals is deregulated. In 1989, Kaufman found this deregulation in two of three HIV-positive hemophiliac boys. It was this study that suggested the daily rise and fall of HGH levels may be what's responsible for its powerful effects on the body. It is this rise and fall that appears to be absent in individuals with HIV.[53]

Thus, raising the circulating levels of HGH and simulating its rise and fall could have a positive effect on AIDS patients. Tests evaluating the effects of hormone replacement on AIDS patients have already begun, and they are showing positive results.

HGH has been shown to be most beneficial in treating HIV-related wasting. AIDS wasting, similar to the wasting that occurs in the undernourished elderly population, is defined as an involuntary weight loss of at least 10 percent of the normal body weight. Wasting occurs when the body starts to use the muscle to fuel biological processes, rather than burning the stores of fat. The sufferer is significantly weakened and vulnerable to deadly infections. It is estimated that wasting is a significant factor in 90 percent of AIDS-related deaths.

We have already discussed HGH's role in helping to build lean body mass. Researchers at the University of Illinois in Urbana tested the influence of HGH on malnutrition recovery in rats. Pregnant rats were given only 60 percent of the amount of food the control group received, so that pups were malnourished at birth, weighing only 62 percent of the control body weight. The pups that were re-fed and given HGH experienced a greater weight gain than those who were

---

53 Jospe N, Powell KR. "Growth hormone deficiency in an 8-year-old girl with human immunodeficiency virus infection." *Pediatrics* 86(2):309–312, 1990.

Laue L, Pizzo PA, Butler K, Cutler GB Jr. "Growth and neuroendocrine dysfunction in children with acquired immunodeficiency syndrome." *J Pediatr* 117(4):541–545, 1990.

Kaufman FR, Gomperts ED. "Growth failure in boys with hemophilia and HIV infection." *Am J Pediatr Hematol Oncol* 11(3):292–294, 1989.

only re-fed. HGH also increased spleen, kidney, and muscle weight.[54]

The effects of malnutrition are similar to the effects of wasting, so it makes sense that HGH should have a positive effect on AIDS patients as well. In a study published in the fall of 1996, Dr. Morris Schambelan and colleagues at UC San Francisco and San Francisco General Hospital tested HGH treatment in 178 patients with AIDS wasting syndrome. It was a twelve-week, placebo-controlled study testing for changes in body composition and aerobic output. The results were such that researchers concluded HGH therapy was the first treatment for wasting syndrome that has been proven to consistently restore lean body mass.

AIDS patients accepted for the study had lost an average of 14 percent of their ideal body weight and had to be able to eat at least 75 percent of their estimated caloric requirements. Ninety of the subjects received daily injections of HGH, while eighty-eight patients received a placebo. At the end of three months, the patients receiving HGH had gained an average of three-and-a-half pounds. This was the net result of an average gain of 6.6 pounds of lean muscle mass and a loss of 3.1 pounds of body fat. These patients also showed an increase of 13 percent in work capacity as measured by treadmill performance. The patients on placebo showed no change in weight, and only a 2 percent improvement in treadmill performance. Some patients on extended treatment eventually gained more than twenty pounds.

Gaining lean muscle mass is the key in preventing the devastation of AIDS-related wasting. The data from the UCSF

---

54 Zhao X, Unterman TG, Donovan SM. "Human growth hormone but not human insulin-like growth factor-1 enhances recovery from neonatal malnutrition in rats." *J Nutr* 125(5):1316–1327, 1995.

study indicates that HGH treatment could play a major role in encouraging this healthy weight gain. "Our study demonstrates that there are therapies that can correct or reverse the loss of lean tissue in patients with HIV-associated wasting," Schambelan said. "Other therapies, such as appetite stimulants, can cause weight gain but have not been as successful in restoring lean tissue."[55]

AIDS patients who have used HGH indicate that they have found new hope. They are stronger, able to do more to take care of themselves, and able to participate more in the activities they enjoy. Much more study still needs to be done in this field, but even if HGH can't cure AIDS, it is still a valuable treatment because it has been shown to significantly improve the quality of life for individuals suffering from late-stage AIDS wasting.

The body of research on the effects of HGH that we have presented here is impressive. We have used the key of HGH to open doors to human health and antiaging that have always been thought to be barred and chained. The more we learn, the more doors we open, and the more mysteries of health we can unlock.

---

55 Mulligan K, Grunfeld C, Hellerstein MK, et al. "Anabolic effects of recombinant human growth hormone in patients with wasting associated with human immunodeficiency virus infection." *J Clin Endocrin Metab* 77(4):956–962, 1993.

CHAPTER 9

HGH, IGF-1, and Cancer

CANCER: INCREASED RISK OR NEW HOPE?

With any new treatment, and especially any new *hormone* treatment, one of the greatest fears is the risk of cancer. This fear has been greater with the development of hormone replacement because of the history of estrogen therapy in post-menopausal women. In past decades, as the number of women using hormone replacement therapy rose, estrogen was linked to an increase in the occurrence of breast and uterine cancer. Testosterone use has also been shown to raise the risk of prostate cancer.

However, we've learned much from these and subsequent studies. Estrogen is now paired with its natural partner, progesterone, and the risk of cancer has all but disappeared. Likewise, lower, balanced doses of testosterone, coupled with anti-prostatic cancer hormones like melatonin and thymus, have almost eliminated the risk of prostate cancer.

EARLY STUDIES

Some very early in vitro studies (studies conducted in petri dishes, outside of the body) indicated that HGH could promote the replication of cancer cells. But as we discussed previously, subsequent studies have proven that this fear is completely unfounded. The human body has an elaborate immune system that does not exist outside the body. In fact, the evidence is strong that HGH could be used in conjunction with cancer treatments to improve the health of patients by strengthening the immune system and improving the overall quality of life.

A CAREFUL LOOK AT CANCER

Simply say the word *cancer*, and we get scared. Cancer research has progressed incredibly in recent years, and the knowledge is always increasing. But the concept of this disease that eats away at the body during years of progressive fatigue and illness is still simply terrifying. Some treatments seem to work to fight cancer, but it is a disease so often associated with death that the uneducated public is not greatly reassured. As a result, anything that even hints at being a cause of cancer is absolutely avoided. Because HGH controls cell division and growth, there has been speculation that HGH therapy would cause cancer, or encourage existing cancer cells to multiply and spread at an even faster rate. Since this is a serious threat and not one to be dismissed lightly, there have been several studies aimed at finding out the truth about any relation between HGH and cancer.

A study by D. Bartlett and associates tested the effect of HGH on tumor-bearing rats. They found that HGH treatment did not increase the size of the tumor or cause the cancer to spread. In fact, the hormone inhibited tumor growth. A similar study from the University of Pennsylvania School of Medicine also showed that HGH inhibited cancerous tumor growth. Research in France, conducted with 5,546 patients over the course of thirty-one years (1959–1990), found that HGH therapy caused no increase in the number of cases of leukemia, lymphoma, or malignancies. Another study from Japan showed that "HGH-receiving patients have normal mutation frequency, regardless of total doses of HGH."[56]

Another study, reported in the April 1985 issue of the *American Journal of Diseases of Children* by S. A. Arslanian, involved thirty-four children with brain tumors. Ninety-four percent of the patients were HGH-deficient after cancer therapy that did not include radiation treatment, and half of this group received HGH as part of their recovery treatment. The HGH group had a lower incidence of tumor recurrence, causing the researchers to conclude that HGH therapy was not associated with an increased rate of tumor growth or recurrence.[57]

Perhaps one of the most balanced assessments of HGH treatment and cancer was offered by Dr. E. Martin Ritzen of the Karolinska Hospital in Sweden, in his study of whether HGH increased the risk of malignancies. He reported, "During the estimated one hundred fifty thousand patient-years of HGH treatment between 1988 and 1992, the incidence of malignancies has been the same as or lower than that of the general population."

In study after study, including those conducted at the Palm Springs Life Extension Institute, authors have concluded that HGH treatment has not contributed to the development of new tumors. Indeed, a number of studies have indicated that HGH therapy can be a beneficial treatment for cancer patients.

---

56 Lin YW, Kubota M, Akiyama Y, et al. "Measurement of mutation frequency at the HPRT locus in peripheral lymphocytes. Is this a good method to evaluate a cancer risk in pediatric patients?" *Adv Exp Med Biol* 431:681–686, 1998.

57 Arslanian SA, Becker DJ, Lee PA, et al. "Growth hormone therapy and tumor recurrence. Findings in children with brain neoplasms and hypopituitarism." *Am J Dis Child* 138(4):347–350, 1985.

Cancer cells develop in healthy people every day, but the immune system usually neutralizes them before they can do us any harm. You cannot talk about cancer without talking about immunity, and HGH enhances immunity. Again, the key is prevention, and growth hormone, by strengthening the immune system, can help prevent cancer cells from ever spreading and becoming a problem.

HGH can also play a role in treating people who have already developed cancer. While it has not yet been proven that HGH can fight cancer directly, we do know that HGH therapy strengthens all the body's systems and organs. The two animal studies mentioned earlier also indicated that HGH caused an increase in overall muscle strength through the course of the disease. This strength means an improved quality of life for cancer victims, specifically those who, because of the disease, are malnourished.

THE PALM SPRINGS STUDY AND THE CANCER QUESTIONS

The alleged increase in incidence of cancer, or the threat of HGH speeding the rate of cancerous growth if already present, has been a major concern in the media. As part of a larger study on our patients' self-assessment of their improvements in health and well-being, the Palm springs Life Extension Institute sent out questionnaires to one thousand patients. On it we included the following questions about cancer:

1. Did you have cancer, any form of cancer, before you entered the study?
2. Have you had any cancer diagnosed since being on growth hormone replacement therapy?

If the answer to either question is yes, please specify the type of cancer.

The majority of the one thousand patients were between the ages of forty and seventy. The minimum age was thirty years for men and twenty-seven years for women. At the other extreme, the oldest man was eighty-two and the oldest woman was seventy-eight.

Seven percent of the one thousand patients, a total of twenty-nine, said they had had cancer in some form before they entered the growth hormone replacement program. (It must be clear to you at this point that we do not consider the presence of cancer a contraindication to growth hormone replacement therapy. In fact, growth hormone replacement therapy may actually become an adjunct therapy for cancer at some time in the future because it boosts one's immunities.)

Of those patients who had growth hormone replacement therapy for six months or longer (the mean being eight months), four of them (approximately 0.97%) developed newly diagnosed cancer. Of the four who developed new cancer during the hormone replacement therapy, two developed squamous cell carcinoma of the skin, and both had had high exposure to sunlight (UV light).

The third one had a squamous cell cancer of the tonsil, and the fourth had plasma cell cancer, which she developed one month after hormone replacement therapy. We do not think anyone can say for sure that this was caused or was in any way due to growth hormone replacement therapy because of the short period of time in which it occurred after she started therapy. Plasma cell disease is a bone marrow type of cancer, and it is extremely unlikely that one month of growth hormone treatment could have produced bone marrow changes. Bone marrow cells take three months to enter peripheral circulation. If you look at the incidence and prevalence of plasma cell disease/cancer in one thousand patients, we do not think you can say this has any relationship to growth hormone replacement therapy.

ACTUAL RATES LOWER

Since some researchers have been concerned that growth hormone could cause undetected cancer cells to divide more rapidly, this statement by Dr. Cass Terry of the Medical College of Wisconsin is significant: "You would think that with more than eight hundred people over the age of forty, that given the normal incidence rate of cancer, some of these people would get cancer. It could be that there is some sort of protective effect from growth hormone replacement. Even more compelling, the level of prostate specific antigen (PSA) levels, a marker of prostate problems, including cancer, did not increase among any of the male patients."

In one amazing case at the Palm Springs Life Extension Institute, we actually saw a severe condition of prostate cancer go into remission after the patient was put on HGH replacement therapy. The individual came to us with prostate specific antigen (PSA) levels of fifty to sixty (healthy PSA levels are zero to four, and cancerous levels range from ten to twenty). After the HGH therapy, the man's PSA levels miraculously dropped to the healthy three to seven range.

"It is mind-boggling," says Dr. Terry, who admits that he does not know why this apparent remission occurred. I speculated that the growth hormone stimulated the immune system, including the natural killer cells, which effectively destroyed the cancer cells.

CONCLUSION

We do not think there is any evidence to show an increase in incidence of cancer related to growth hormone replacement therapy. In fact, we believe that the overall strengthening of the cells, organs, systems, and immunities, which HGH typically brings, reduces the rate of cancer. If higher levels of HGH were responsible for increases in cancer, we would see a higher incidence of cancer in young people and a lower incidence in older people. This, of course, is exactly the opposite of real life statistics.

CHAPTER 10

How to Use the Power of HGH

STRONGER MEDICINE

While telomerase or its analogs may not be available to us in any usable form for another ten to twenty years, HGH is not something you can pick up with your eggs and diet soda at the grocery store, either. Obtaining and using HGH is a little more difficult than ordering a super-duper slicer-dicer-chopper-mixer, and there are no operators standing by waiting to take your credit card number. HGH is a potent prescription medication that should only be used under the supervision of an experienced physician, and only after blood tests establish your current hormone levels. HGH is most effective when it is replaced only to the levels we see in young adults. Both too little and too much HGH can be detrimental to your health.

We would like to tell you that you can raise your remaining HGH production to young adult levels with proper exercise, adequate sleep, and a balanced diet, but we can't. These things will boost HGH production slightly, but the stimulated HGH secretion will likely not be sufficient to counter the debilitating and degenerative effects of aging. We all know people who are active and have had healthy habits throughout their lives. They may be aging at a slightly slower rate than people who are not taking care of themselves, but while they work hard at living properly, they still eventually experience the symptoms of age-related HGH deficiency.

Because of the incredible benefits that HGH therapy can bring, researchers and marketers are developing products and supplements that will stimulate the pituitary to release more HGH. Many of these products are already available at health food stores, by mail, or on the internet. Some of these products are controversial, some are ineffective, and some do produce some change in HGH levels. But you should remember that if it's real HGH, it has to be prescribed by a physician. If you can get it without a prescription, it's not real HGH.

HGH RELEASERS: MAGIC BULLETS?

Let's take a look at all the practices and products that are known to stimulate HGH secretion. Growth hormone releasers, or secretogogues, include exercise, sleep, nutrients, hormones, and certain medications.

Exercise

Exercise, particularly intense anaerobic exercise like weightlifting, is one way to stimulate HGH secretion. Studies have shown that this resistance training provokes an acute increase in the circulating levels of HGH. This could be one of the reasons for the increase in energy that people experience when they exercise. To ensure optimal HGH levels with or without HGH therapy, weight training two to three times a week is a good idea.

Sleep

Adequate sleep is also important because of the nocturnal release of HGH. Remember when you were a child and your parents told you that you only grow while you're asleep? Turns out there was some truth to what they said. Research has indicated that the largest amount of HGH is normally released in a peak that occurs about two hours after the onset of deep sleep, typically at about 1:00 a.m. If you are going to depend on sleep to help boost your HGH levels, you need to be in bed and deeply asleep by 11:00 p.m.

Growth Hormone Releasing Drugs

L-dihydroxyphenylalanine, also known as L-dopa, is a prescription medication that is one of the best-known growth hormone releasers. In the United States, it is FDA-approved for the treatment of neurological diseases, namely Parkinson's disease. L-dopa, however, is an amino acid precursor to several fundamental neurotransmitters that control the functioning of the pituitary gland, so it is also an effective HGH releaser.

A 1982 study used L-dopa on aging rats. The treatment increased the mean plasma and pituitary HGH concentrations and improved the amplitude of HGH pulses. The older rats treated with L-dopa showed HGH pulses and levels equivalent to those of young rats.[58]

In 1990, a study by J. W. Pritchett used L-dopa to treat patients with very serious and debilitating long bone fractures. L-dopa was presumed to stimulate the release of HGH, and the theory was that higher levels of HGH would be helpful in bone

---

58 Sonntag WE, Forman LJ, Miki N, et al. "L-dopa restores amplitude of growth hormone pulses in old male rats to that observed in young male rats." *Neuroendocrinology* 34(3):163–168, 1982.

growth and repair. After six months, 84 percent of the patients had full movement and use of their fractured limbs and experienced no pain. This recovery suggests that the HGH-releasing properties of L-dopa greatly improve the speed and quality of healing in seriously fractured bones.[59]

Researchers, and those who have used L-dopa as an antiaging drug, report very positive results. This is still a powerful prescription drug, however, with some negative side effects when overdosed.

GHB—gamma-hydroxybutyrate—is another HGH releaser that should only be taken under the direction of a physician. GHB is a precursor to gamma-amino butyric acid (GABA) which acts as a neurotransmitter in the central nervous system, and as a pituitary stimulator. Along with stimulating the release of HGH, GHB also calms, relaxes, and induces sleep. Bodybuilders and other users swear by the powerful and dramatic effect of GHB on their levels of HGH. They also report that GHB greatly enhances the libido.

GHB was widely available over-the-counter in health food stores in the 1980s. During the 1990s, it gained popularity as a recreational drug. In 1990, the FDA banned the sale of GHB in the United States. Although its possession has not yet been declared a federal crime, several states have outlawed it. While safe if taken in appropriate doses under medical supervision, GHB has the potential for serious side effects if taken in large amounts or with alcohol.

Diet and Dietary Supplements

Certain foods that are part of a normal, healthy diet can also prompt the pituitary to release more HGH. The dietary key to HGH release seems to be adequate amino acid and carbohydrate

---

59 Pritchett JW. "L-dopa in the treatment of nonunited fractures." *Clin Orthop* 255:293–300, 1990.

intake, but some of the B vitamins, including B3 (niacin) and B6, have also been identified as HGH releasers.

Amino acids are probably the most effective and the most popular HGH releasers. Amino acids are the building blocks that the body uses to construct the proteins that become part of muscle, bone, tissue, and several of the hormones. Most of the amino acids are naturally present in our body, or we can get them from the foods we eat. Researchers have isolated specific amino acids that appear to stimulate the release of HGH from the pituitary. By taking supplemental amino acids, you can raise your serum HGH levels somewhat, but not to the twenty-year-old level, which is our goal.

Arginine is probably the most widely used and widely accepted amino acid HGH releaser. In fact, one study showed that oral arginine supplements produced greater increases in HGH production than did treatment with L-dopa.[60] Arginine is taken as a single amino acid or in combination with other substances to boost HGH levels. One of the major drawbacks to arginine use is that, in order to see any benefits, an individual has to take more than eight grams of the amino acid each day. This is especially difficult because arginine has a rather unpleasant taste.

Lysine joined with arginine is one of the most common amino acid combinations. The amino acid lysine is an essential protein building block, and the addition of lysine improves the overall HGH-releasing properties of arginine. It also helps increase IGF-1 metabolism, and boosts the immune system by stimulating thymic hormone secretion. On its own, lysine fights herpes and cold sores, and helps in recovery from surgery and injuries by aiding in the formation of collagen.

---

60 Isidori A, Lo Monaco A, Cappa M. "A study of growth hormone release in man after oral administration of amino acids." *Curr Med Res Opin* 7:475–481, 1981.

Ornithine is another amino acid commonly combined with arginine to stimulate the release of HGH. In fact, arginine is a precursor to ornithine. For this reason, ornithine performs many of the same functions mentioned in our discussion of arginine.

Another of the most common forms of ornithine supplementation is ornithine alpha-ketoglutarate, or OKG. This is a combination of ornithine and the precursor of another amino acid, glutamine. These two substances paired increase HGH levels more than ornithine alone. By also promoting the production of glutamine, users get a further exercise benefit of increased endurance and decreased muscle fatigue.

Glutamine is the most abundant amino acid in the body. It also becomes a potent brain booster when converted to glutamic acid. Partly because of this ability to stimulate the brain, glutamine also induces the secretion of HGH.

Glycine, a lesser-known amino acid, is often found in combinations with arginine and ornithine. A Japanese study showed that glycine alone could also be a powerful HGH releaser. The study reported that subjects who received oral glycine supplements had a 10 times greater hormone secretion than those in the placebo group.[61]

Tryptophan, like L-dopa and GHB, is a neurotransmitter precursor. In the brain, this amino acid converts to serotonin, which has a calming effect and helps treat stress, anxiety, and depression. It is also used to treat migraine headaches. Tryptophan stimulates HGH release directly with its effect on the pituitary gland, and also by treating insomnia. By helping a user sleep, tryptophan can return the body to its regular sleep patterns, thereby promoting the healthy, natural, nocturnal release of

---

61 Kasai K, Kobayashi M, Shimoda S. "Stimulatory effects of oral glycine on human growth hormone secretion." *Metab* 27(2):201–208, 1978.

HGH. Although tryptophan has a long history of safe use, in December 1989 the FDA reported more than six hundred cases of a flu-like syndrome associated with a blood abnormality in those taking the amino acid. Although the problem was traced to a contaminated batch from a single manufacturer, tryptophan is no longer available in the United States in supplement form.

Carnitine is commonly thought of as a weight-loss aid. That is because this amino acid prevents fatty acid buildup by transporting longchain fatty acids to the muscle, where they can be burned and used as energy. But carnitine also works as a growth hormone releaser, because it increases the declining number of glucocorticoid receptors in the hippocampus, the site of negative feedback between the pituitary and adrenal glands. The age-related decline in the glucocorticoid receptors is believed to be related to neuroendocrine aging, which includes the drop in HGH production. By stimulating production of glucocorticoid receptors, carnitine slows down the aging of the entire neuroendocrine system.

Tyrosine is the amino acid precursor to the neurotransmitter dopamine. A lack of dopamine leads to depression, poor immune functions and, most importantly, a depressed secretion of HGH. So by keeping enough dopamine in the brain, tyrosine stimulates the release of HGH.

NOT SO MAGIC

Amino acid supplements and other HGH-releasing products and practices generally have the benefit of being cheap and convenient. However, HGH releasers are still not the perfect solution. Supporters of secretogogue use claim that amino acids are a more natural way to bring HGH levels up. But many of these natural substances, when taken in large amounts, cause serious side effects and still cannot stimulate HGH enough to bring it to the levels we desire for antiaging purposes (an IGF-1 level of 280 to 350).

Some of the most common side effects include nausea and diarrhea. Some amino acids can cause damage to the liver. Generally, these only occur with improper administration, but because these amino acids have other jobs in the body in addition to the stimulation of the pituitary gland, there is always a chance of negative physical responses. In most of the inexpensive and popular over-the-counter formulas, the probability is that an HGH releaser will not work adequately.

Growth hormone releasers, most of which are taken orally, have to pass through the liver before they can be used by the body, so patients with liver problems should avoid this avenue of treatment. Also, because these substances must pass through the digestive system before they can get into the bloodstream to reach the pituitary gland, it is more difficult to control the actual timing of HGH release. This is a serious drawback, because timing the release of HGH is almost as important as having enough HGH in your system. As we know, the peak of HGH secretion occurs during sleep, which may be the primary characteristic responsible for HGH's amazing effects on the body.

Depending on your body composition, age, and even what you've eaten during the day, HGH releasers could be telling your pituitary to release too little HGH, or none at all. Insufficient HGH release means you will not see all of the growth and restoring benefits of optimum HGH blood levels. In fact, some studies show that only very high doses of amino acids stimulate the release of HGH. Despite the fact that these substances are generally available and easy to use, they should not be self-prescribed. As mentioned earlier, each amino acid has a critical dosing point, under which it may not stimulate sufficient HGH release, and over which it could cause side effects. A doctor can recommend the safest and most effective dosages, and only a physician can monitor HGH blood levels to guarantee that they are high enough to be beneficial to your antiaging efforts.

IF YOU ARE OVER 50

If you are over fifty, natural HGH releasers will probably have no effect whatsoever on you. In many cases, the decline in HGH levels in the body is not just a result of the pituitary failing to release the hormone. It is more often caused by the pituitary gland deteriorating and not being able to even produce the hormone anymore. Studies with HGH releasers indicate that the older you get, the less effective amino acids or pituitary-stimulating drugs will be on your pituitary gland. With an aging pituitary, you will have to take large amounts of any releaser to prompt any secretion of HGH. Even with maximum doses of secretogogues, many in the older population don't see much benefit because they are still unable to bring their HGH levels anywhere close to the optimum.

The reason has less to do with the efficacy of the amino acid-growth hormone relationship and more to do with the simple fact that the pituitary gland is older. In these cases, the releasers are telling the gland to do something it no longer can do. Supplying the basic amino acid building blocks to an aged pituitary gland is as ineffective as putting high-octane fuel in an old, rusted car to make it perform like a new, souped-up sports car. It is like trying to pump water out of a dry well. You'll wear yourself out pumping and still end up with an empty bucket.

A SHOT IN THE NIGHT: THE BEST SOLUTION

The absolute best way to make sure your body is functioning with optimal levels of HGH is to control HGH levels directly, by injection. A single molecule of HGH is made up of a chain of 191 amino acids, which makes it, molecularly speaking, a very large hormone. The size of the HGH molecule limits the number of ways to get it into the body. Other hormones that are made up of smaller molecules are generally taken orally as pills or transdermally, through the skin.

However, with HGH, the digestive process is too destructive and breaks down the molecule into smaller pieces, changing the overall composition and rendering the hormone useless. Other hormone supplements can be applied to the skin in a gel form, and from there they are absorbed into the blood vessels of the skin, and carried to the rest of the body. This method would not work with HGH because of its large molecular size. If applied to the body in cream or gel form, the precious HGH can never get into the dermal blood vessels because it is too large to pass through the layers of skin.

Small injections are the solution to the problem of how to get this vital hormone into the areas where it can do the most good. The form of HGH administration that uses the same type of insulin syringes that diabetic patients use is virtually painless. It is also a very simple process, and with only minimal training, patients learn how to give themselves the treatment, making it a very convenient therapy.

In addition to convenience, there are many other powerful benefits to this method of HGH replacement. As mentioned earlier, replacement, rather than stimulation, is the only way to make sure that many people, especially those over fifty, can bring their hormone levels to the optimal levels of the twenty-year-old. Injection is also the quickest way to get the hormone into your system and working for your health.

Subcutaneous injection in the thigh area is the method of choice because of its more physiologic rate of absorption, when compared to intravenous or intramuscular injection. The subcutaneous technique involves getting the hormone underneath the skin and into an area of capillary activity. The hormone can then be picked up by the blood and taken to the parts of the body that need it.

This is important, because it allows us to most closely mimic the body's natural cycles and patterns. With recombinant HGH, we already have an identical copy of the HGH that is in the body. Now we just need to get it to the organs and target tissues at a time when they are used to receiving and using it. As mentioned before, HGH is released in pulses and not a continuous stream. The largest pulse comes at night, during REM sleep. We have discovered that by injecting the hormone right before bed, we can closely imitate the natural sleep-release cycle of a young, healthy pituitary gland. The closer we can get to reproducing the natural or physiological functions of a healthy body, the more we eliminate the chance of any negative side effects. Similarly, the benefits are much faster and stronger with a physiologic approach to replacement.

MINIMIZING SIDE EFFECTS

In their enthusiasm for improved health, many people believe that if a little of something is good, then a lot must be better. When we talk about HGH therapy, a lot can be much worse than a little. Many things are unhealthy if taken in excess. Any of the medicines or supplements you buy at your local supermarket can be dangerous if you take too much. This is why manufacturers provide recommended dosing guidelines.

Even natural supplements like vitamins, minerals, and herbal combinations come with cautions about taking too much. Red meat, in and of itself, is not a toxic substance, but consuming excessive amounts can raise your uric acid levels and increase your risk of high cholesterol, heart problems, and gout. Even something as delicious as chocolate will make you sick if you have too much at once. None of these substances is bad in and of itself, and many help us maintain health, but any one of them taken in excess will have negative side effects. As with cold medicine or aspirin, HGH can also be harmful if it is not taken properly and in the recommended amounts.

Much of the fear of negative side effects from HGH replacement is a result of early testing with the hormone using high-dose (eighteen to thirty-two units a week) and low-frequency (three times a week) applications. These studies noted raised blood sugar, joint pain and swelling, and some incidence of carpal tunnel syndrome. Medicine is an ever-evolving field, and the results of every study, whether positive or negative, help us to learn more about our bodies and what we can do to keep them healthy. In the case of HGH, the positive outcomes of early tests gave researchers great hope and enough promise to keep studying and testing the benefits of hormone replacement. Any negative side effects of treatment then became the subject of subsequent testing to determine how to make the therapy even safer. Over the years and as a result of these many tests, we now know how to minimize, and in most cases eliminate, side effects entirely. Other tests have also proven that fears about some previously conjectured or reported side effects are completely unfounded.

Hyperglycemia: Passing Fancy

Early tests with HGH replacement noted the occurrence of raised blood sugar or glucose levels, a condition known as hyperglycemia. This lasted two to three hours after a large dose of HGH was administered. It does not occur in our low-dose method, which usually consists of 0.8 to 1.3 units per injection. In most cases, especially those involving patients who had no history of diabetes, this was a temporary phenomenon lasting anywhere from three to six months. Also, as we mentioned in our earlier discussion of diabetes, HGH therapy can actually benefit the diabetic patient by increasing the body's sensitivity to insulin. This means that a diabetic patient will eventually require smaller amounts of insulin to keep a healthy balance in the body.

So the temporary rise in blood sugar levels certainly does not eliminate diabetic patients from taking advantage of the benefits of HGH therapy. It simply means that these patients must be monitored very closely to assure that blood sugar levels never get to a dangerous level during the first three to four months of treatment. This supervision would also indicate if and when a change in insulin doses would be appropriate.

Fluid Retention: Water, Water Everywhere

Another common side effect of early high-dose, low-frequency HGH therapy was fluid retention that caused mild edema, or swelling. Left unchecked, this led to minor joint pain and a low incidence of carpal tunnel syndrome. However, joint pain and carpel tunnel syndrome rarely show up as a result of our low-dose, high-frequency method. They can be eliminated in the very few who do experience this side effect by further lowering the dose.

Fluid retention can also be a concern for patients with congestive heart failure. In this condition, the heart can no longer meet the demands of the body. In extreme cases, patients with congestive heart failure can develop pulmonary edema, or excessive fluid in the lung tissue. Like diabetics, patients with congestive heart failure should be closely monitored but can still greatly benefit from the program, especially the heart-strengthening qualities of HGH.

A DOSE-DEPENDENT NATURAL BALANCE

Many of the fears about HGH replacement have proven to be unfounded, and negative side effects virtually disappear with proper dosing. In our studies at the Palm Springs Life Extension Institute, we have developed a treatment program that drastically reduces the chance for any negative side effects. We monitor our patients and all their levels very closely for negative results. If there are any minor problems, the dose of HGH is adjusted down, and the symptoms disappear. Based on a questionnaire filled out by 282 patients from the Palm Springs Life Extension Institute, the side effects of HGH replacement therapy were negligible. Fewer than 5 percent reported fluid retention, and there was only a 2 percent occurrence of joint pain and a 1.77 percent incidence of carpal tunnel symptoms.

Approximately 4 percent developed acne, and 2 percent had unwanted hair growth. One percent reported prostatitis, two respondents noted the occurrence of oily skin, and only one patient developed an increase in blood sugar. All of these symptoms, in this particular group, may have been related to concomitant testosterone replacement therapy rather than HGH.

Again, the key is to mimic the body's natural functions. With any medical treatment, this is a major issue. The more natural or similar the new organ, blood, or hormone is to that which was in the body previously, the better the chance that the body will accept the addition.

HOW OFTEN?

In the early HGH replacement studies, this natural approach was not considered, and doses of the hormone were given only three times a week. This procedure was based on the standard administration of HGH in children, when the supply of HGH was still very scarce and only administered in a hospital setting.

During normal secreting activities, the serum HGH pattern is characterized by high nocturnal levels, starting one to two hours after the onset of sleep. Other secretions during the day are much less predictable and consist of smaller bursts, but we do need daily secretions of HGH to keep the body functioning at its healthy peak.

Our bodies are not accustomed to, or equipped for, handling large doses of HGH only three times a week, just as eating small meals more often would be better than eating three large meals three times a week. Besides, the pituitary gland does not secrete HGH just three times a week. If we give HGH three times a week, we would get some of the benefits of the hormone, but we would have to suffer some of the same negative side effects observed by Dr. Rudman in his landmark 1990 study and described on previous pages.

A more recent study by Maxine Papadakis and colleagues at the University of California in San Francisco employed the identical high-dose, low-frequency method of administration that Dr. Rudman used in his study. Not surprisingly, the Papadakis research revealed a 77 percent incidence of negative side effects, such as swelling and joint pain. When the dose was reduced by up to 50 percent, these negative side effects "disappeared or remitted markedly within two weeks."[62]

Appendix D shows the results of a large study of growth hormone-deficient patients treated with the low-dose, high-frequency methods used at the Palm Springs Life Extension Institute.

---

62 Papadakis MA, Grady D, Black D, et al. "Growth hormone replacement in healthy older men improves body composition but not functional ability." *Ann Int Med* 124(8):708–716, 1996.

DAILY DOSING IMPROVES RESULTS

In our studies at the Palm Springs Life Extension Institute, daily dosing improved the positive results of HGH therapy and increased the overall benefits. The growing body of research and clinical data indicates that the more closely administration can mirror the body's natural secretion rhythms, the more effective the treatment will be. A shot before bed allows the hormone to enter the bloodstream and peak at physiologic levels, at approximately the same time naturally secreted HGH reaches its peak. Another dose upon waking imitates the lesser daytime secretion of HGH. Because we don't want the pituitary to shut down entirely, our treatment includes dosing with HGH for only six days a week. A seventh day without replacement therapy ensures that the pituitary doesn't get lazy about producing endogenous HGH.

OTHERS FOLLOW THE LOW-DOSE, HIGH-FREQUENCY LEAD

Large doses, combined with less frequent administration, are the major cause of the unpleasant side effects researchers have observed. Because of this, a number of study centers have reduced their doses of the hormone. For example, Johns-Hopkins University initiated their study with a dose of 30 ug/kg of the patient's body weight, given three times a week at approximately 8:00 p.m. Because the high-dose, low-frequency method tends to cause water retention and carpal tunnel syndrome, Johns-Hopkins reduced its dose to 20 ug/kg. Likewise, the University of Washington, which initiated treatment at 24 ug/kg, reduced its dose to 12 ug/kg.

Several other studies have proven the safety and effectiveness of the low-dose, high-frequency method of HGH administration. Three different studies, ranging in duration from two to twelve months, all used low-dose HGH administration on fifty subjects.

The studies reported that the subjects experienced a decrease in body mass and cholesterol, increase in lean muscle mass and bone mass density, and improvement in exercise capacity. Impressively, in all three of these low-dose, high-frequency tests, no adverse side effects were reported.[63]

HOW MUCH IS ENOUGH?

Getting the proper dosage of HGH can be a bit tricky. Again, this is powerful medicine and should not be tampered with by those who don't know what they're doing. Unlike aspirin or cold medicine, we can't slap a label on the side of a bottle of HGH advising the average adult how much to take. Because we each have a slightly different body composition and varying physical needs, there is no standard prescription for HGH. The key to combating side effects is to determine what is most beneficial for each patient. This requires a knowledgeable physician and individualized dosage requirements.

Now acknowledged by mainstream medicine as a specific syndrome, adult growth hormone deficiency is being recognized and treated more frequently, giving rise to increased opportunity to study the effects of long-term growth hormone replacement. Several such studies published recently tracked and reported on

---

63 Russell-Jones DL, Weissberger AH, Bowes SB, et al. "Protein metabolism in growth hormone deficiency, and effects of growth hormone replacement therapy." *Acta Endocrinol* 128 Suppl 2:44–47, 1993.

Russell-Jones DL, Weissberger AH, Bowes SB, et al. "The effects of growth hormone on protein metabolism in adult growth hormone deficient patients." *Clin Endocrinol* 38:427–431, 1993.

Russell-Jones DL, Weissberger AH, Bowes SB, et al. "The effect of growth hormone replacement on serum lipid, lipoproteins, apolipoproteins and cholesterol precursors in adult growth hormone deficiency patients." *Clin Endocrinol* 41:345–350, 1994.

those taking human growth hormone for periods as long as thirty-six months.[64]

These studies unanimously concluded that growth hormone treatment restores lean body mass, reduces fat mass, increases bone mass, improves protein synthesis, increases hydration of the body, and improves exercise capacity. It was also lauded for improving psychological well-being, including energy, sleep, and emotions. One study even reported that sick leave days and hospitalizations decreased about 50 percent after test subjects had taken human growth hormone for six months or more.[65]

NO MAJOR SIDE EFFECTS

To date, we have not had any major side effects, including carpal tunnel syndrome, in our series of patients. There have been no

---

64 Christ ER, Carroll PV, et al. "The consequences of growth hormone deficiency in adulthood, and the effects of growth hormone replacement." *Schweiz Med Wochenschr* 127(35): 1440–1449, 30 Aug 1997.

Meling TR, Nylen ES. "Growth hormone deficiency in adults: a review."*Am J Med Sci* 311:153–166, 1996.

65 Verhelst J, Abs R, et al. "Two years of replacement therapy in adults with growth hormone deficiency." *Clin Endocrinol (Oxf)* 47(4):485–494, 1997.

Nass R, et al. "Effect of growth hormone replacement therapy on physical work capacity and cardiac and pulmonary function in patients with growth hormone deficiency acquired in adulthood." *J Clin Endocrinol Metab* 80:552–557, 1995.

Nass R, Strasburger CJ. "Effects of growth hormone treatment on serum lipids and lipoproteins in adults with growth hormone deficiency." *Eur J Endocrinol* 130 Suppl 2:34, 1994.

O'Halloran DJ, Tsatsoulis A, Whitehouse RW, et al. "Increased bone density after recombinant human growth hormone (GH) therapy in adults with isolated GH deficiency." *J Clin Endocrinol Metab* 76:1344–1348, 1993.

Laursen T, et al. "Metabolic effects of growth hormone administered subcutaneously once or twice daily to growth hormone deficient adults." *Clin Endocrinol (Oxf)* 41(3):337–343, 1994.

reported cases of cancer, and prostate specific antigen (PSA) levels in male patients have not increased. Our results are in agreement with and extend those of Dr. Rudman. We are continuing to monitor the effects of HGH replacement therapy on blood cholesterol, triglycerides, HDL, LDL, PSA, blood pressure, and cardiovascular fitness. Please see Appendix E for an in-depth study of the effects of low-dose, high-frequency HGH treatment.

The low-dose, high-frequency method of administration used at the Palm Springs Life Extension Institute seems to be the safest and the most effective method to date. It has consistently produced only one very minor side effect in certain patients: some adults on our program indicate experiencing mild pain, limited swelling, and periodic itching at the site of the injection. These reactions generally cause little concern and resolve themselves within a day or two. The other side effects mentioned earlier in this chapter do not appear at all when HGH is administered in a natural, physiological way. Patients experience all the benefits of HGH without suffering any pain or discomfort, because they are receiving just the right amount of the hormone.

It has maintained my weight, I have the energy that I had twenty years ago, and it has made me want to go out and exercise. —Jacque B., patient of the Palm Springs Life Extension Institute

CHAPTER 11

~

HGH Contraindications and Abuse

ADULTS TREATMENT IS NOT RECOMMENDED FOR

While all existing research has demonstrated that HGH therapy is extremely safe, we have identified some people who should not take HGH. Other than for the following four patient populations, HGH is a safe treatment, and there are seldom any reasons to deny a patient HGH replacement therapy and all the benefits it provides.

Those who should not take HGH without an extensive medical evaluation include patients who have at any time suffered from gigantism or acromegaly; those with a history of severe, untreated carpal tunnel syndrome; patients with pituitary adenoma, a benign tumor that can cause excessive secretion of HGH; and those with certain types of active cancer.

ABUSE BY BODY BUILDERS AND ATHLETES

Another group who should not take HGH includes those who want to take large amounts of HGH just to bulk up. This is not only unwise, it is also illegal; using HGH simply for body building purposes is a federal offense. The benefits of HGH therapy, especially its ability to increase muscle mass, are so obvious that abusing the power of HGH is a temptation for some. Unfortunately, no matter how much evidence is presented to show the dangers of overdosing and abusing the hormone, there will always be some who will push treatment limits for a perceived physical gain. We want to make it clear that abuse of the hormone is dangerous, and though we strongly recommend using the hormone to treat HGH deficiency, we do not approve of or condone the use of growth hormone for those who simply want to bulk up or boost physical ability in sports.

HGH therapy is not designed to create a race of superhumans who will be able to leap tall buildings in a single bound. Our goal for you is optimum health. People who abuse the hormone simply for its performance-enhancing abilities are not doing themselves any favors. Abusers are often competition athletes or bodybuilders who use doses that are one hundred times the medically recommended dose. These doses may result in increased muscle mass, but such unnatural levels of the hormone mean an increase in all the negative side effects we have already discussed. HGH abuse greatly increases your risk of encountering dangerous and potentially life threatening physical problems.

ACROMEGALY CAUSED BY ABUSE

Post-puberty HGH abuse can lead to acromegaly, or abnormal growth in parts of the body, such as the hands, toes, skull, and nose. Symptoms of acromegaly include prominent cheekbones, a protruding jaw, rough skin, an increase in body hair, and enlarged nose, lips, tongue, and forehead. Abusive amounts of HGH also stimulate excessive cartilage growth, causing significant joint pain. Although acromegaly sufferers are often quite tall, HGH abuse will not lead to increased stature, because after the teenage years, the bony growth centers have already fused. In other words, in post-adolescents, there can be no more increase in height, no matter how much of the hormone is taken.

OTHER HEALTH CONCERNS FOR ABUSERS

Even more seriously, HGH abuse greatly increases the chance for cardiac failure. This is partly due to the increase in heart size, often leading to congestive heart failure. Acromegalic adults, for example, experience a very high mortality rate, and most ultimately die of cardiac failure—50 percent by age fifty, and 89 percent by age sixty. In addition, HGH abuse can lead to diabetes, impotence, and an increased incidence of osteoporosis.

Despite these well-documented results and their accompanying cautions, the abuse of HGH continues to increase. Abusers are willing to do anything to look good, be muscular, and win. For these people, the potential for dangerous side effects that may cause serious health problems even decades after use has been discontinued does not outweigh the benefits of winning.

The irony is that while acromegalic adults often appear to be muscular and strong, they actually end up being quite weak. As time goes on, they suffer from myopathy, an abnormality of the muscle tissue. This causes the muscles themselves to lose their mass and strength. The gains are short-lived and the dangers much, much too great to ever justify HGH abuse.

USING HGH RESPONSIBLY

Multiple studies have proven that if an individual does not abuse HGH, the healthy benefits he or she receives are incredible, and the side effects are virtually non-existent. Drs. Rowen, Johannsson,

Johannsson, and Bengtsson of the University Hospital of Goteborg, Sweden, had this to say in a 1995 article: "When one does not abuse or overdose HGH, there is simply no evidence suggesting that HGH replacement therapy causes any long-term side effects."

The abuse by some uninformed and careless individuals should in no way discourage the research and treatment of HGH deficiency. Human growth hormone, when used properly, can energize, strengthen, and improve the patient's emotional well-being and overall quality of life. It is a powerful tool that, like so much in life, can be used for good, or can be abused. The key to proper use is finding a treatment method that most closely mimics the body's physiologic functions, and seeking the goal of ultimate health, rather than ultimate physical power.

CHAPTER 12

~

Total Hormone Gene Therapy

THE ENTIRE ORCHESTRA

We have discussed in some detail the great benefits of HGH, but as you learned in earlier chapters, this is not the only hormone that keeps our bodies healthy. The benefits of HGH are magnified when the other hormones are functioning at their optimal levels.

Earlier, we compared the power of HGH to the hand controlling the actions of a marionette. The hand gives the puppet life and largely determines the quality of the overall performance. But what if some of the strings connecting the hand to the puppet were broken or weak? Some movements would be impossible, and others wouldn't be nearly as smooth as desired. The strings are the other hormones in the body. HGH can accomplish incredible things by itself, but when the other hormones are also at their optimal levels, the power of HGH is even greater.

In the body, the hormones all work together to keep our cells, and thereby our organs, functioning well. The hormones that the pituitary releases (one of which is HGH) then trigger other glands, telling them to release their hormone. Because of this interconnectedness, the declining levels of one hormone will undoubtedly affect the others, causing their levels to drop as well. As we have seen, disturbing the delicate balance between hormones causes our health to deteriorate. The drop in all hormone levels, and the accompanying health problems, are a main characteristic of the aging body.

Replacing the hormones reverses those characteristics, and any hormone you replace will invariably influence the other hormones and their functions. Because of this influence, replacing all the hormones simultaneously is important to ensure the safety of any hormone therapy. For example, earlier we mentioned the increased risk of breast and uterine cancer with estrogen replacement therapy for post-menopausal women. In recent years, however, estrogen has been combined with its natural partner, progesterone, and the risk of developing cancer from hormone therapy has almost entirely disappeared.

We want hormone replacement to be as natural as possible. As tests and experience have proven, estrogen doesn't work alone in the female body. Neither does HGH play out its important role in our physical health by itself. Our ultimate goal is to restore the youthful balance of hormones that exist in a young, healthy body.

Replacing the hormones is also essential in maintaining the health of the telomeres, which tell the cells to keep rebuilding. As we discussed earlier, the telomerase gene appears to respond to high levels of hormones by producing telomerase, which in turn prompts cell rejuvenation. It is for this reason that we have termed this treatment Total Hormone Gene Therapy.

In order to replace all the hormones effectively, you need a doctor's involvement. This is partly because some hormones, such as HGH, are only available with a prescription, but also because a doctor's supervision is even more important to help guarantee you are getting the most out of your treatment, and that you aren't getting too much of any one hormone. (The OTC versions of so called "HGH" are fakes because the law requires all real HGH to be sold under prescription. One only need to ask for the transaction to be carried out in the presence of a police officer to know if the HGH is real or fake. If it is real, the seller will be arrested for selling the prescription drug OTC).

Remember, we only want to replace hormones to their optimal levels and not beyond. Because each hormone affects all of the others, there is the potential for one to cause the hypersecretion of another, resulting in possible negative side effects. A total hormone gene therapy program, prescribed and monitored by a physician, can anticipate and treat these problems. Even though many of the hormones, such as DHEA and melatonin, are available without a prescription, we strongly caution you to use them only under a doctor's supervision. As with everything else in life, these hormones can offer tremendous benefits, but inappropriate use can increase the potential for negative side effects.

With that caution, let's learn about the various hormones and their benefits.

DHEA

Flip the pages of any health and fitness magazine, or browse the Internet, and you will find hundreds of ads for DHEA (dehydroepiandrosterone), the antiaging hormone that distributors claim will turn your life around. It has been proven to energize the body; restore sex drive; improve memory; lower blood cholesterol; fight obesity, heart disease, and stress; and strengthen the immune system. People who take DHEA say they look and feel years younger.

DHEA is one of the latest crazes in antiaging medicine, and since it was approved by the FDA for sale as a nutritional supplement, hundreds of manufacturers have sprung up claiming that their blend is the most natural and most pure, yielding the greatest benefit. Some companies have even developed test kits for determining your own DHEA levels without having to see a doctor. DHEA has become big business.

Of course, not all this enthusiasm is unwarranted. The results of DHEA testing prove that it is a very important hormone. DHEA, which is produced in the brain and in the adrenal cortex, is the most abundant hormone in the body and is a precursor to the sex hormones. Levels of DHEA reach their peak around age 30 and then decline steadily as we age. Dr. Norman Shealy, in his book *DHEA: The Youth and Health Hormone*, notes that low levels of DHEA can be linked to almost every major disease. Levels are low in cases of obesity, diabetes, immune deficiencies, cancer, high blood pressure, and heart disease. The theory, then, is that by replacing DHEA levels, we can battle these diseases and maintain health for a longer period of time.[66]

Increased HGH Production

The benefits of DHEA replacement may sound similar to those received through HGH therapy. An explanation of this similarity can be found in the results of a 1994 test which studied the effects of DHEA treatment on the overall health of thirteen men and seventeen women, ages forty to seventy. The majority of hormone recipients reported a vast improvement in mood and energy, but even more impressive was the effect of DHEA replacement on the subjects' HGH levels. The study reported that restoring DHEA

66 Shealy NC. *DHEA: The Youth and Health Hormone*. New Canaan: Keats Publishing, Inc., 1996.

to youthful levels in elderly men and women greatly increased the blood levels of IGF-1.[67]

This protein, you will remember, is a product of HGH secretion, and the levels of IGF-1 give us an accurate measure of the amount of HGH in the body. Therefore, DHEA can increase the levels of HGH, which may partly account for the all-encompassing, powerful effects of DHEA treatment.

Improved Sexual Function

One of the most common reports with DHEA use is improved sexual function. This is also a result of DHEA affecting other hormones. In fact, DHEA is often referred to as a mother hormone because DHEA is a precursor to the sex hormones. DHEA treatment can help raise the levels of testosterone, estrogen, and progesterone to youthful amounts. As we know, these hormones are directly responsible for the body's sexual operation and sexual pleasure. By supplementing DHEA and raising the levels of the sex hormones, sexual function, including erection, lubrication, and orgasm, is improved.

Weight Loss and Muscle Gain

Another common report from those who supplement DHEA is that they lose weight and gain muscle. One study showed the link between DHEA and obesity in rats, as those who were treated with the hormone gained less weight and had a lower body fat even though they ate the same food as the control group. In humans, another study reported a 31 percent reduction in body fat percentage in approximately one month. Some statistics have also shown that

67 Morales AJ, Nolan JJ, Nelson JC, Yen SS. "Effects of replacement dose of dehydroepiandrosterone in men and women of advancing age." *J Clin Endocrin Metab* 78(6):1360–1367, 1994.

DHEA works as an appetite suppressant. But no matter how it works, the evidence is clear: DHEA helps regulate body weight and body fat, ensuring that they are at healthy levels.[68]

Brain Power

This powerful hormone also has a strong influence on the functioning of the brain. This is because there is more DHEA in the tissue of the brain than in any other tissue in the body. Optimal DHEA levels improve memory and mental acuity. This can be explained by a study by Eugene Roberts, who added DHEA to brain tissue of mice. He observed that the addition of DHEA activated the growth of inter-neuron connectors. The more of these connectors there are in the brain, the quicker the communication and transfer of information between brain cells.[69]

The number of neural connectors also influences memory. One common memory test used with mice is the maze. Healthy mice who find their way through a maze once can remember the correct path on subsequent trips through the maze. However, older mice repeatedly have much greater difficulty negotiating the maze on subsequent trips than the young mice, indicating an age-related memory impairment. In one study, after older mice were given DHEA supplements, they were able to function just as well in the maze as the younger mice.

The benefits of DHEA are certainly not limited to mice. In two separate studies, elderly patients who were suffering from depression and memory problems were treated with DHEA.

---

68 Cleary MP. "The antiobesity effect of dehydroepiandrosterone in rats." *Proc Soc Exp Biol Med* 196(1):8–16, 1991.

69 Roberts G. "DHEA and its sulfate (DHEAS) as neural facilitators: effects on brain tissue in culture and on memory in young and old mice." *The Biologic Role of Dehydroepiandrosterone (DHEA).* Kalimi M, Regelson W, eds. New York: Walter de Gruyter, 1990.

After four weeks of treatment, most of the depression was gone, and the subjects showed dramatic improvements in semantic and incidental memory, the two types of memory to deteriorate first in those who suffer from Alzheimer's. DHEA may prove to be a powerful therapy, not only for treating Alzheimer's, but for preventing it, too.[70]

Heart Health

Optimal levels of DHEA are also very important in maintaining heart health. Elizabeth Barrett-Connor, of the University of San Diego, published a study in 1986 showing the relationship between DHEA levels and heart disease. In her study of 242 men over age fifty, she reported that those with high levels of DHEA had half the incidence of heart disease as those with low levels. Because of these powerful results, she also concluded that DHEA seems to help prolong life even in patients with no history of heart disease.[71]

Immunity

This life-extending quality could be attributed to DHEA's effect on the immune system. In virtually every case of immune deficiency disease, the sufferer is DHEA deficient. Replacing DHEA enhances the creation of antibodies. This could be one explanation for DHEA's ability to inhibit tumor initiation, as

---

70 Wolkowitz OM, Reus VI, Roberts E, et al. "Antidepressant and cognition-enhancing effects of DHEA in major depression." *Ann NY Acad Sci* 774:337–339, 1995.

Wolkowitz OM, Reus VI, Roberts E, et al. "Dehydroepiandrosterone (DHEA) treatment of depression." *Biol Psychiatry* 41(3):311–318, 1997.

71 Barrett-Connor E, Khaw KT, Yen SS. "A prospective study of dehydroepiandrosterone sulfate, mortality and cardiovascular disease." *N Eng J Med* 315(24):1519–1524, 1986.

found in a 1993 study testing DHEA's cancer-fighting abilities in rats and mice.[72]

This immune power also affects diseases like AIDS. In an article in the *Journal of Infectious Diseases* (November 1991), researcher William Regelson reported that only when DHEA levels drop do people with HIV develop full-blown AIDS. In fact, low DHEA levels indicated twice the risk of HIV patients developing AIDS.

Control of Stress Hormones

One of the ways DHEA boosts the immune system is by controlling the production of the stress hormones cortisol and adrenaline. Stress hormones are released by the adrenal glands, and they raise blood sugar and increase the heart rate in order to prepare the body to cope with whatever is causing the stress. Ideally, all of these hormones are used up in dealing with the stressor, usually in physical output. But when they are not used up—when we internalize the stress and cannot act on it physically—the stress hormones accumulate in the body. With an unhealthy buildup of stress hormones, our body's immune response is inhibited, and T-cells, which normally fight off infections, don't work as well as they should. The end result is that we become more susceptible to illness.

This is not really news to most of us. We've been hearing for years how many common illnesses, as well as serious diseases, develop as the result of stress. In fact, if you don't feel well, most likely someone will tell you that your ailment is a result of all the stress in your life, and that you'd get well if you could just relax more. But how many of us can really get rid of all the stress that

72 Schwartz AG, Pashko LL. "Cancer chemoprevention with the adrenocortical steroid dehydroepiandrosterone and structural analogs." *J Cell Biochem Supp*. 17G:73–79, 1993.

we face each day? With jobs, traffic, families, financial pressures, and the evening news, stress is as regular a part of our lives as sleeping and eating. For many people, it is just not possible to cut out all the pressures they deal with each day. So the key is to manage and deal with the stress effectively. Exercise is a great way to do this. Trying not to internalize the stress is also helpful.

Another effective way to counter the effects of stress in our lives is to make sure our DHEA levels are optimal. Studies indicate that when our stress levels rise, our DHEA levels drop. Replacing the DHEA helps to neutralize or control the stress hormones. A 1980 study by Drs. William Regelson and Vernon Riley tested the power of DHEA to counter the damaging effects of stress. Previous studies by Riley had indicated that extreme stress could kill mice. He also established the link between stress and a shrunken thymus gland, as all the mice that died from the stress had abnormally small thymus glands. In the Regelson and Riley study, they recreated the same stresses, but this time gave the mice DHEA. In these cases, despite the severe, life-threatening stress, the thymus remained strong, and the mice remained basically healthy.[73]

Other studies examining the effect of DHEA on auto-immune diseases such as lupus and multiple sclerosis report that, though high levels of DHEA cannot cure the diseases, the hormone does seem to be able to greatly improve the quality of life of these patients.[74]

---

73 Regelson W, Coleman C. *The Superhormone Promise.* New York: Simon and Schuster, 1996.

74 van Vollenhoven RF, Morabito LM, Engleman EG, McGuire JL. "Treatment of systemic lupus erythematosus with dehydroepiandrosterone: 50 patients treated up to 12 months." *J Rheumatol* 25(2):285–289, 1998.

Kalimi M, Regelson W, eds. *The Biologic Role of Dehydroepiandrosterone.* New York: Walter de Gruyter, 1990.

Few Side Effects

One reason all of these results are so impressive, and that the FDA approved DHEA as a nutritional supplement, is the very low occurrence of negative side effects reported with DHEA use. Because it is a precursor to the sex hormones, primarily testosterone, DHEA can have androgenic or testosterone-like effects on women, causing increased facial hair, menstrual changes, and acne. Some users have also reported mood changes and increased aggression. Some male patients have experienced nasal congestion and mild insomnia. There are also cases of enlarged prostate that we've encountered with self-prescribed, excessive DHEA users who have come to the Palm Springs Life Extension Institute. Generally, though, these side effects occur only when the dosage is much too high.

PREGNENOLONE

If DHEA is the mother hormone, pregnenolone is the grandmother, because it is the precursor to DHEA. Like DHEA, pregnenolone is produced in the brain, where it is found in high concentrations, and in the adrenal glands. Like most hormones in the body, pregnenolone production declines dramatically with age.

Increased DHEA Levels

We've talked here about the benefits of DHEA supplementation. Because pregnenolone is a hormone precursor, it raises the blood levels of DHEA and other cholesterol hormones such as testosterone and estrogen.

Pregnenolone is a powerful hormone on its own. While most of the other hormones focus on the body's physical needs, pregnenolone caters to our mental needs and is essential for keeping our brain functioning at its peak capacity.

Pregnenolone, which is found in higher concentration in the brain than in any other organ, serves to enhance our mental functions. It also is a powerful influence for improving the transmission of nerve impulses. Most notably, pregnenolone fights mental fatigue, improves memory, relieves depression, and enhances mood. These functions of pregnenolone have been studied for over fifty years, with impressive results.

Two studies conducted in the 1940s by the same research team demonstrated the brain-boosting power of pregnenolone. The first study tested the mental skills of pilots and non-pilots on a flight simulator. While learning to fly, some of the subjects were given pregnenolone, while the others received a placebo. The results, after two weeks of testing, showed that regardless of previous flight training, those who received the hormone did substantially better with flight simulation than did those in the placebo group.

The second study tested the effects of pregnenolone on factory workers who were paid by the piece. Generally, these were leather cutters, lathe operators, and optical workers. The results showed an increase in total productivity, fewer errors and waste, and a higher-quality finished product from workers who were given pregnenolone. The participants in this study also reported an increase in energy, decrease in fatigue, improved mood, and better ability to cope with stress. This study suggests that pregnenolone can not only improve mental acuity but can also control stress and prevent fatigue. Because of these mood-enhancing abilities, pregnenolone has been effective in treating depression and in maintaining emotional well-being.[75]

---

75 Pincus G, Hoagland H. "Effects of administered pregnenolone on fatiguing psychomotor performances." *J Aviat Med* 15:98–115, 1944.
Pincus G, Hoagland H. "Effects of industrial production of the administration of delta 5 pregnenolone to factory workers." *J Psychosomatic Med* 7:342–346, 1945.

A more recent study brought to light just how powerful a mental stimulant pregnenolone is. Drs. John E. Morley, James F. Flood, and researcher Eugene Roberts studied the effects of several hormones on the learning and memory abilities of rats. Researchers taught the rats the route through a maze. Then the rats were given either DHEA, pregnenolone, or testosterone. To test the effect of the hormones on memory, the rats ran the maze again one week later. The pregnenolone-treated rats greatly outperformed even those that were given the other hormones, and this performance was achieved using unbelievably small doses of pregnenolone. The dramatic results of this test and the human tests from the 1940s earned pregnenolone the title of most powerful memory enhancer—up to one hundred times more powerful than other hormones.[76]

Pregnenolone and Alzheimer's Disease

Positive discoveries have led to current studies, including several evaluating the potential of pregnenolone to treat Alzheimer's disease. Many people believe pregnenolone could be effective in treating even full-blown Alzheimer's disease, because studies have shown that Alzheimer's patients have much lower levels of the hormone than healthy individuals of a similar age. Pregnenolone may also aid in Alzheimer's treatment because it is a precursor to estrogen and progesterone which, in recent

---

76 Flood JF, Morley JE, Roberts E. "Pregnenolone sulfate enhances post-training memory processes when injected in very low doses into limbic system structures: the amygdala is by far the most sensitive." *Proc Natl Acad Sci USA* 92(23):10806–10810, 1995.

Flood JF, Morley JE, Roberts E. "Memory-enhancing effects in male mice of pregnenolone and steroids metabolically derived from it." *Proc Natl Acad Sci USA* 89(5):1567–1571, 1992.

years, have been shown to help prevent the onset of this terrible disease.[77]

Early Use for Arthritis

Before pregnenolone was ever tested for its mental enhancement abilities, it was widely used to treat the pain of arthritis. In the 1930s and '40s, individuals who suffered from rheumatoid arthritis reported that they experienced much less pain, greater energy and strength, and improved mobility when they took pregnenolone. It was a safe and effective treatment, with virtually no side effects reported even after years of continual use. It also appeared to be a powerful therapy for other disorders, such as osteoarthritis, scleroderma, and psoriasis.

But in the late 1940s, pharmacies introduced the drug cortisone, which brought users almost immediate relief from arthritis pain, as opposed to the slower response of a week or more with pregnenolone. With pharmaceutical companies promoting cortisone, pregnenolone treatment was eventually forgotten. Cortisone was later found to have serious side effects. Though pregnenolone has not since been widely used to treat arthritis and joint pain, the great success of the earlier use indicates that hormone replacement would be an effective and safe therapy for arthritis sufferers.[78]

---

77 Roberts E. "Pregnenolone—From Selye to Alzheimer and a model of the pregnenolone sulfate binding site on the GABAA receptor." *Biochem Pharmacol* 49(1):1–16, 1995.

78 Freeman H, Pincus G, et al. "Therapeutic efficacy of delta 5 pregnenolone in rheumatoid arthritis." *J Am Med Assoc* 143:338–344, 1950.

Davison R, Koets P, Snow WG, Gabrielson LG. "Effects of delta 5 pregnenolone in rheumatoid arthritis." *Arch Int Med* 85:365–388, 1950.

Pregnenolone Use in Other Diseases and Injuries

We are still learning so much about this hormone and its powers. Recently, researchers have begun to see possible applications for pregnenolone therapy in the treatment of conditions like multiple sclerosis, spinal cord injuries, cardiovascular problems, and for boosting the immune system and strengthening the skin. Among the most impressive studies is one indicating that pregnenolone may aid in repairing the myelin sheath, a fatty layer that protects the nerves, to prevent multiple sclerosis. Another study at the College of William and Mary analyzed the effect of pregnenolone on rats that had suffered severe spinal cord injuries that often result in paralysis. A surprising majority of the rats that were treated with the hormone were able to stand or walk in three weeks, and a few regained much of their pre-injury ability.[79]

The Grandmother Role

Part of the reason pregnenolone has such a powerful effect on so many areas of the body is its grandmotherly role. As pregnenolone levels increase, typically so will those of DHEA and the sex hormones. This is part of what allows pregnenolone to improve overall physical and mental health. Recent studies have shown that male and female bodies use pregnenolone differently. Given the same amounts of the hormone and the same tests, results vary by gender. The conclusion from these studies is that in women, more of the pregnenolone becomes estrogen, while men use more pregnenolone to make testosterone. Pregnenolone treatment appears to be completely safe, but we have already shown that too much DHEA, estrogen, or testosterone in the body can cause

---

79 Guth L, Zhang Z, Roberts E. "Key role for pregnenolone in combination therapy that promotes recovery after spinal cord injury." *Proc Natl Acad Sci USA* 91(12):308–312, 1994.

some unpleasant side effects. If your physician monitors not only your pregnenolone levels but all your hormone levels, you can safely enjoy the benefits of increased mental acuity, better memory, and a greater sense of well-being.

ESTROGEN

One of the strongest arguments for careful, total hormone gene therapy comes from our experiences with estrogen. As pioneers in hormone replacement therapy, estrogen taught us a lot about how hormones work together and the importance of balancing and replacing all the body's hormones, instead of just one.

Estrogen is primarily a female hormone, but is also found in small amounts in men. In women, estrogen is produced in the ovaries and the adrenal glands. The production and secretion of estrogen is controlled by the hypothalamus, which works with the pituitary and pineal glands to control sexual development, a process in which estrogen plays a major role. In women, estrogen is what stimulates ovulation each month and prepares the lining of the uterus to accept the egg if fertilized. It is also responsible for physical maturation, including the filling out of the breasts and hips, and development of the female reproductive organs during puberty.

Help for Menopausal Symptoms

Because of its definitive role in the female reproductive system, estrogen has been prescribed for more than forty years to help women who experience severe hot flashes and other extreme menopausal symptoms. Menopause occurs when the ovaries no longer produce estrogen and the other main female hormone, progesterone. Hormone replacement gives women relief from the sweating, fatigue, vaginal dryness, depression, and decreased libido that are traditionally part of menopause and may last for years. Women also reported that the estrogen therapy improved their skin and muscle quality, as well as their mental outlook.

In addition, estrogen therapy was found to decrease the incidence of osteoporosis and heart disease, so women continued taking the hormone after menopause. These wonderful results prompted physicians to prescribe estrogen therapy to almost any woman going through menopause, even those who did not experience extreme symptoms. Estrogen therapy seemed to be the wonder treatment.

The Case for Hormone Balancing

The wonder treatment unfortunately proved to have a serious drawback. Women who used estrogen replacement continually for several years had a much higher risk of developing endometrial (uterine) and breast cancers. A report from the National Cancer Institute showed that women who took estrogen had a 50 percent greater risk of developing breast cancer than women who had never used the hormone. Another study reported that women who had taken estrogen had a two- to eight-times increased risk of getting endometrial cancer. One explanation for this phenomenon is that, as part of the normal menstrual cycle, estrogen stimulates the build-up of uterine tissue. During menstruation, the buildup decreases. But since post-menopausal women no longer experience normal menstrual cycles, the supplemental estrogen-induced buildup of the uterus lining goes unchecked, putting them in danger of uterine cancer.

The increased risk of breast and uterine cancer led researchers to seek treatment methods that would still yield the great benefits of estrogen therapy without increasing the incidence of cancer. The key to estrogen therapy, as with so much in medicine, is to mimic the body's natural functions. No matter what a woman's age, estrogen works with other hormones to maintain optimum physical and mental health. In a healthy body, estrogen works most closely with progesterone, another of the sex hormones. Researchers found that when women were given progesterone along with the estrogen, the risk of breast and uterine cancer virtually disappeared.[80]

Adding Other Hormones Eliminates Risks

Recently we've discovered that the risk of cancer is reduced even more by adding DHEA and HGH to the treatment. So by making estrogen part of a total hormone gene therapy program, we can safely and more effectively gain the many long-term benefits of estrogen therapy. Because of the long history of estrogen use, we now have a great deal of clinical data outlining just what estrogen does for the body. Along with relieving menopausal symptoms, studies show that estrogen greatly reduces the risk of osteoporosis and heart disease, improves brain function, fights against the effects of aging, and increases the average life expectancy of users.

Osteoporosis

Women are at greatest risk for developing osteoporosis, which afflicts one in four females over age sixty, and 50 percent of all people seventy-five and older. This supports the theory that estrogen can be used to treat the disease. What we've seen with estrogen users is that estrogen, though not a cure for osteoporosis, does slow down the rate of bone loss, preserving a woman's strength and mobility. Studies show that women who take estrogen have a 25 percent reduction in bone loss

80 Gambrell RD, Maier RC, Sanders BI. "Decreased incidence of breast cancer in post-menopausal estrogen-progestogen users." *Obstet Gynecol* 62(4):435–443, 1983.

and only 25 percent of the number of hip fractures as women who do not take estrogen. Spinal fractures are also decreased by 50 percent. Additionally, women on estrogen have stronger teeth and fewer dentures. In fact, the hormone reduces tooth loss by 50 percent. Some of these effects may be, at least in part, because estrogen induces the release of HGH, which in turn stimulates bone production.

REDUCING HEART DISEASE

Estrogen also plays an important role in dramatically reducing the chance of developing heart disease, including heart attack, stroke, heart failure, and arrhythmia. Heart disease is rare in younger women, but the incidence increases threefold during the post-menopausal years, accounting for approximately 30 percent of the deaths in women over age fifty. This incredible leap in heart disease cases prompted researchers to make the connection between the rise in heart disease and the decline in estrogen levels.[81]

The link holds true, as women who use estrogen have half the risk of developing heart disease. Estrogen has been shown to strengthen both the heart muscles and the blood vessels, and lower LDL cholesterol levels while raising HDL levels. These benefits also mean that estrogen can significantly help women who already have heart disease. A stronger heart means longer life.

STAYING YOUNGER

Not only can estrogen give women longer life, but because of its antiaging benefits, estrogen also helps them have a *younger* life. Many women, after using estrogen to help reduce menopausal symptoms,

---

81 Schwartz J, Freeman R, Frishman W. "Clinical pharmacology of estrogens: cardiovascular actions and cardioprotective benefits of replacement therapy in post-menopausal women." *J Clin Pharmacol* 35(1): 1–16, 35(3):314–329, Jan, Mar 1995.

stay on the hormone because it helps them look and feel younger. Estrogen boosts energy levels, increases libido, strengthens hair, and improves the quality of skin, resulting in fewer wrinkles. Many of these actions can be attributed to estrogen's antioxidant properties. Estrogen, like vitamin E and beta-carotene, acts as a scavenger in the body, neutralizing the free radicals that destroy cells. Free radical destruction often shows up as thin, wrinkled skin.

WHAT ESTROGEN CAN DO FOR YOUR BRAIN

Almost more important than what estrogen can do for your body is what it can do for your brain. We used to believe estrogen had a significant influence only on the body systems below the neck. However, the discovery of estrogen receptors in the brain changed that view. These receptors tell us that estrogen influences very specific functions of the brain, and the number of receptors could explain why women's brains seem to work differently than men's. This could be the reason fluctuating hormone levels can have such a powerful effect on mood and why one of the symptoms of menopause is depression. Women on estrogen therapy reported an overall increase in mood and a greater sense of well-being.[82]

The Alzheimer's Association estimates that four million Americans have Alzheimer's disease, and statistics show that it is three times more common in women than in men. The first clue that researchers had into estrogen's influence on the brain was the fact that women who had used estrogen were less likely to develop Alzheimer's disease.[83] A study of more than

82 Sherwin BB. "Sex hormones and psychological functioning in post-menopausal women." *Exp Gerontol* 29:423–430, 1994.

83 Tang MX, Jacobs D, Stern Y, et al. "Effect of oestrogen during menopause on risk and age at onset of Alzheimer's disease." *Lancet* 348:429–432, 1996.

two thousand women at the University of Southern California showed that long-time estrogen users were 40 percent less likely to develop Alzheimer's disease than women who had never used the hormone.

Another study from Columbia-Presbyterian Medical Center reported in the August 17, 1996 issue of *Lancet*, that the risk of Alzheimer's disease decreased 5 percent each year that a woman took estrogen. This five-year study of women ages seventy and older also showed that estrogen users who developed Alzheimer's did so much later than women who had never taken the hormone. Dr. Richard Mayeux of Columbia University says that it may be impossible to entirely prevent Alzheimer's in certain people, but that the hormone seems to be able to delay the onset of the disease by five years or more. Even these few years will greatly improve the patient's quality of life. By decreasing the number of Alzheimer's cases, estrogen therapy could greatly reduce the cost of treating Alzheimer's disease, which is currently estimated at more than sixty-seven billion dollars a year.

Research also suggests that although estrogen is not a cure, patients with Alzheimer's can be treated with the hormone to improve their current condition. This treatment would be effective because estrogen is involved in the formation and protection of brain cells, and it indirectly triggers the production of a key neurotransmitter that is essential to the memory functions of our brains. In fact, estrogen has been proven to sharpen and improve memory in healthy individuals as well.

A recent study by Dr. R. Schmidt of Austria indicated that women on estrogen replacement therapy performed better on neuropsychological tests than women who had never taken the hormone. Schmidt went one step further and performed MRIs on the test subjects. Amazingly, the women who had taken estrogen supplements showed much less age-related brain tissue damage than the control group.[84]

Thus, not only can estrogen enhance brain functions such as memory, it can protect the precious cells of the body's most complex organ. A report from Johns Hopkins shows that estrogen also protects the brain from damage caused by a stroke. After researchers induced strokes in both male and female rats, results showed that males suffered three times more brain damage than females. The test was performed again using female rats who had had their ovaries removed so they were not producing normal amounts of estrogen. The females then had brain damage equal to that of the males. Researchers concluded that estrogen protected the cells by creating a way for blood to get past the blockage and into the brain.

The Life-Prolonging Effects of Estrogen

By keeping the brain, the bones, and especially the heart healthy, estrogen also prolongs life. A report published in the January 1, 1996 edition of the *Journal of Obstetrics and Gynecology* outlined just what a difference estrogen can make on overall life expectancy. Dr. Bruce Ettinger, head of the research team, looked at the medical histories of 454 women born between 1900 and 1915. All of the women were part of the Kaiser Permanente Medical Care Program in Oakland, California, and approximately half had used estrogen at some point in their lives, while the other half never had. Among the estrogen users, mortality was decreased by an amazing 46 percent. Ettinger attributed most of this to the decreased incidence of heart attack and stroke. In fact, coronary

84 Schmidt R, Fazekas F, Reinhart B, et al. "Estrogen replacement therapy in older women: a neuropsychological and brain MRI study." *J Am Geriatr Soc* 44(11):1307–1313, 1996.

heart disease was reduced by 60 percent, and strokes by an amazing 70 percent in the women of the estrogen group, who also showed a decreased incidence of lung cancer. This study, and others, suggests that estrogen therapy could increase the overall life expectancy of women by two to three years![85]

Dr. Ettinger is quick to point out, though, that these are the benefits of long-term estrogen therapy. Many women who start taking estrogen do so to manage their menopausal symptoms. But women should not stop using estrogen when hormonal symptoms disappear. Each year a woman is on the treatment, her chances of getting heart disease or Alzheimer's decrease and her chances of living even longer increase.

But estrogen does more than help women live longer. When balanced with progesterone, estrogen makes both mind and body stronger, helping women live *better.*[86]

PROGESTERONE

As we have discussed, estrogen therapy alone is insufficient for women who want to attain optimal health. In the female body, estrogen works very closely with progesterone to regulate the menstrual cycle and the female hormonal responses. In more than forty years of use, we have witnessed the power of estrogen. We are just now beginning to understand the equally incredible power of progesterone.[87]

---

85 Ettinger B, Friedman GD, Bush T, Quesenberry CP, Jr. "Reduced mortality associated with long-term post-menopausal estrogen therapy." *Obstet Gynecol* 87(1):6–12, Jan 1996.

86 Zubialde JP, Lawler F, Clemenson N. "Estimated gains in life expectancy with use of post-menopausal estrogen therapy: a decision analysis." *J Fam Prac* 36:271–289, 1993.

87 Lee JR. *Natural Progesterone: The Multiple Roles of a Remarkable Hormone.* Sebastopol, Calif.: BLL Publishing, 1993.

Progesterone is produced in the corpus luteum (the follicle that ruptures during ovulation), the adrenal glands, and in the placenta during pregnancy. This hormone plays a major role in the menstrual cycle as it prepares the uterine lining to accept the egg if it is fertilized. If there is no fertilization, progesterone levels drop, triggering the sloughing off of the lining of the uterus. Progesterone is also vital to a healthy pregnancy and is produced in large amounts in the placenta. Without sufficient progesterone in her system, a woman has a difficult time carrying her pregnancy to term.[88]

Progesterone and Mood

Progesterone strongly influences mood. It is the low levels of progesterone just before a menstrual period that cause some women to experience what is called PMS, which traditionally includes irritability, moodiness, and physical discomfort. The drop in progesterone triggers a less-than-pleasant emotional response, suggesting that progesterone acts as a natural antidepressant and tranquilizer. In fact, progesterone is often prescribed for women who experience severe moodiness associated with PMS.[89]

ENHANCING ESTROGEN

The levels of progesterone produced every month begin to drop when a woman is in her late thirties. By menopause, the amount of progesterone in the body fluctuates wildly. In fact, much of the menopausal discomfort women experience is due to a lack of balance between estrogen and progesterone levels. So just as

---

88 Dan AJ, Graham EA, Beecher CP, eds. *The Menstrual Cycle*. New York: Springer Publishing Co, 1980.
Puhl JL, Brown CH, eds. *The Menstrual Cycle and Physical Activity*. Champaign, Ill.: Human Kinetics Publishers, Inc, 1986.

89 Weidegger P. *Menstruation and Menopause: The Physiology and Psychology, the Myth and the Reality*. New York: Alfred A. Knopf, 1976.

estrogen alleviates the symptoms of menopause, progesterone also helps eliminate hot flashes and mood swings. Studies show that progesterone enhances estrogen function, including its cardioprotective abilities.[90]

As we discussed earlier, progesterone also protects against endometrial cancer by maintaining the lining of the uterus, preventing cancer cells from attacking uterine tissue.[91]

Sex Drive

On its own, progesterone performs many functions. One of its main jobs is controlling a woman's sex drive. In fact, some people call progesterone the source of a woman's libido. It is the hormone that gives women the enhanced sex drive they sometimes feel during ovulation. Progesterone also aids thyroid action and helps the body use fat for energy rather than store it.

Bone Building

One of the most impressive functions of progesterone is that of bone building. Estrogen has been praised for years as the best prevention against osteoporosis that many people, particularly women, experience as they age. However, two new reports show that progesterone can go one incredible step further than estrogen in preventing osteoporosis.

In our discussion of human growth hormone, we talked a little about the dynamics of bone growth. Old bone cells are continuously being broken down by osteoclasts, while osteoblasts

---

90 PEPI Trial. "Effects of estrogen or estrogen/progestin regimens on heart disease risk factors in post-menopausal women. " *J Am Med Assoc* 273:199–208, 1995.

91 PEPI Trial. "Effects of hormone replacement therapy on endometrial histology in post-menopausal women." *J Am Med Assoc* 275(5):370–375, 1996.

stimulate the production of new, healthy bone cells. Osteoporosis occurs when the osteoclasts take over and bone destruction occurs at a much faster rate than bone growth. In fact, post-menopausal women lose about 2 percent to 4 percent of their bone mass each year. Estrogen has been proven to be able to slow down the destruction, but not stop it altogether.

Dr. Jerilynn C. Prior from the University of British Columbia has been studying the effects of various hormones in both animal and human osteoporosis. Her studies show that progesterone can not only stop bone destruction, but it can also stimulate the osteoblasts to form new bone![92]

This action appears to be entirely independent of the functions of estrogen. Published the same year as the Prior paper was a study by Dr. John R. Lee. For three years, Dr. Lee tested the bone health of one hundred post-menopausal women who were at risk for developing osteoporosis. The women all ate a healthy diet, including calcium supplements, exercised regularly, limited their alcohol consumption, and were instructed not to smoke. All the test subjects took either estrogen and progesterone supplements or the progesterone alone. At the end of the study, well over half of the progesterone-only test group not only demonstrated that bone destruction had slowed, but they also showed an increase in bone density.[93]

Dr. Lee says that it makes sense that progesterone, not estrogen, is responsible for bone health, since bone mass begins decreasing at the same age progesterone levels begin to drop. He believes that with progesterone treatment, the bone thinning damage of osteoporosis can actually be reversed!

---

92 Prior JC. "Progesterone as a bone-trophic hormone." *Endocrine Revs* 11:386–398, 1990.

93 Lee JR. "Is natural progesterone the missing link in osteoporosis prevention and treatment?" *Med Hypotheses* 35(4):316–318, 1991.

As with estrogen, we will probably discover greater and greater benefits the longer progesterone is used. Our experience with progesterone thus far shows that there are virtually no negative side effects. However, optimal health is attained when hormones are at youthful levels, so both progesterone and estrogen should also be prescribed and monitored by a trained physician.

A WORD ABOUT SYNTHETICS AND "DESIGNER" HORMONES

Estrogen has been in use for a long time, and progesterone is now in great demand. As a result, there are many different versions of the hormone available for prescription and purchase. It is important for women to understand the differences between the supplements, so that with the help of a physician they can choose the treatment that will yield the greatest benefits and the least amount of risk.

The most common estrogen prescriptions are for the synthetic (also known as a non-bioidentical hormone) estrogen, Premarin, which is a blend of estrogens found in the urine of pregnant mares. These estrogens are natural for horses, but they are not the same as natural estrogen found in humans and can therefore cause some unpleasant side effects. Some of these negative effects include excessive water retention, headaches, and moodiness.

Similarly, a synthetic progesterone called progestin, or Provera, is most often combined with Premarin in prescription. The prevalence of synthetic chemical hormones is partly due to old habits. Physicians who began prescribing hormones decades ago used synthetics because that was all that was available for oral administration. Today, medical technology allows many hormones to be given orally without being digested by the stomach. And today, many doctors are not even aware of the significant differences between progestin and progesterone, and Premarin and estrogen. Also, the drug companies cannot patent the natural hormones, so they have no incentive to market or promote them. Instead, they pour lots of money into promoting their synthetic designer hormones.

Synthetic hormones are man-made chemicals that do not bear the same molecular structure as the hormones the body naturally produces.

There are natural versions of both estrogen and progesterone available. In order to be called *natural*, these supplements must be molecularly and chemically identical to the hormones found naturally in a healthy body. In natural supplements, there are no foreign, man-made chemicals that the body has never seen before and which may cause negative side effects. Many women, after experiencing some of the negative effects triggered by synthetic hormone use, become frustrated and disillusioned with hormone therapy. Many feel they have to take the hormones in order to prevent heart disease and osteoporosis but hate how the synthetic hormones make them feel. On the other hand, women who take natural hormones report fewer side effects and generally stay on the treatment.

Not only do natural hormones prevent side effects, but because they are identical to the hormones in the body, they do their job better than synthetics. In 1989, Dr. Joel T. Hargrove and associates at Vanderbilt University Medical Center compared the effects of synthetic versus natural hormones. Ten menopausal women took natural supplements, while five more took synthetics. Researchers discovered that the women taking natural hormones showed an even greater reduction in cholesterol levels, with an increase in HDL cholesterol, when compared to the synthetic users. They also reported that at the end of the study, all the women using natural hormones wanted to continue the treatment, while two out of five women on synthetic hormones wanted to call it quits.[94]

Some women have taken synthetic hormones for years and have experienced all the benefits, with no side effects. If this has been your experience with hormone replacement, you should still consider switching to natural hormones, because some studies indicate that the synthetic progesterone does not protect against estrogenic cancers. For thousands of women who may have tried synthetic estrogen and progesterone and just didn't feel well, the option of natural hormones may be the answer. Each woman should discuss her situation with a knowledgeable health care professional, and together they can decide on the best treatment.[95]

TESTOSTERONE

Just the word *testosterone* conjures up images of muscle-bound football players and sex-hungry teenage boys. This way of thinking limits our knowledge of a very important hormone that has been misunderstood for years.

---

94 Hargrove JT, Maxson WS, Wentz AC, Burnett LS. "Menopausal hormone replacement therapy with continuous daily oral micronized estradiol and progesterone." *Obstet Gynecol* 73:606–612, 1989.

95 Mohr PE, Wang DY, Gregory WM, et al. "Serum progesterone and prognosis in operable breast cancer." *Br J Cancer* 73(12):1552–1555, 1996.
Nyholm HC, Christensen IJ, Nielsen AL. "The prognostic significance of progesterone receptor level in endometrial cancer." *Ugeskr Laeger* 159(5):601–604, 1997.
Roy JA, Sawka CA, Pritchard KI. "Hormone replacement therapy in women with breast cancer. Do the risks outweigh the benefits?" *J Clin Oncol* 14(3):997–1006, 1996.
Weiss NS. "Health consequences of short- and long-term post-menopausal hormone therapy." *Clin Chem* 42(8 Pt 2):1342–1344, 1996.

Testosterone is the primary male sex hormone. It is responsible for male sexual development during puberty, and is critical in maintaining erectile function, libido, normal energy levels, and mood. But testosterone controls physical functions all throughout the body—not just those below the belt. It declines, as do the rest of the body's hormones, with age. Some studies indicate that by age eighty, testosterone levels drop to only one-fifth of what they were in youth. Testosterone has been studied for years, but is still, unfortunately, not widely used in hormone replacement.

Our knowledge about testosterone dates back into the mid-1800s when a German physiologist removed the testes of two roosters and transplanted them into two other roosters. The castrated roosters grew fat and lazy while the other two stayed strong and energetic, and their combs, sex organs for roosters, kept on growing. The 1935 Nobel Prize went to a scientist who isolated the testosterone molecule and illustrated the structure. In 1938, another scientist discovered that testosterone had beneficial effects on glucose tolerance, and a year later it was learned that the hormone improved angina pectoris, a pain in the chest caused by some types of heart disease. During World War II, a physician transplanted the testes of a dying soldier into an older soldier who was suffering from gangrene caused by a gunshot wound. With the addition of testosterone in his system, the older soldier quickly recovered. In 1951, it was discovered that testosterone increases lean muscle mass and, almost ten years later, scientists observed that the hormone could also lower cholesterol.

Menopause and Andropause

So why, with this history, is testosterone not used by men who have a hormone deficiency? One study estimates that out of the four to five million American men of all ages with testosterone deficiency, only two hundred fifty thousand receive testosterone replacement. Why is testosterone therapy so far behind estrogen treatment?

One reason may be the nature of andropause, or the male menopause. Many people compare andropause to menopause, but there are some clear differences. When the female menopause occurs, there is a distinct physiological change which announces its arrival: the cessation of menstrual periods. In contrast, there is no obvious physiological event to warn males when andropause has arrived. Testosterone levels begin declining when a man is in his thirties, and at andropause, the hormone drops at a rate of about 1.5 percent per year. While the levels of total testosterone may not drop drastically, the free testosterone, which is the biologically active testosterone, declines dramatically with age.

Though the drop in free testosterone is dramatic, andropause makes itself known physically in a more gradual way. It shows up as a progressive decrease in energy, thinning bones and muscles, increased body fat, depression, and impaired sexual function. Research also links testosterone deficiency with hypertension, obesity, and an increased risk of heart disease. Dr. Jens Moller of Denmark, a pioneer in the field of testosterone replacement, observed that, of the men who showed low levels of testosterone, approximately 80 percent experienced reduced libido and difficulty initiating and maintaining an erection, 92 percent reported a reduced overall sexual satisfaction, 82 percent experienced fatigue, 70 percent reported depression, and approximately 60 percent of the men reported increased irritability, aches, pains, and stiffness.

Another significant difference between andropause and menopause is that andropause can occur anywhere between the ages of thirty and fifty, whereas menopause almost always takes place when a woman is in her late forties or early fifties. Stress can often play a significant role in determining when a man's testosterone levels drop. One of the most profound effects of declining testosterone is impotence, and some studies suggest that a man only lives for about twenty years after becoming impotent. At age fifty, approximately 5 percent of the male population has become impotent. This increases to 27 percent by age seventy, and 75 percent by age eighty. The later in life a man experiences andropause, the longer he'll live, the healthier he'll be, and the longer he'll remain sexually potent.

Testosterone deficiency is a problem that can be corrected.[96] But because of the link between testosterone, sexuality, and the world's perception of manhood, many men are reluctant to talk about andropause or a possible testosterone deficiency. Dr. Adrian S. Dobs of Johns Hopkins University School of Medicine explains that this may be another reason testosterone treatment is so far behind studies with estrogen replacement. "Unfortunately, most men aren't comfortable discussing the symptoms of testosterone deficiency, such as a decrease in sexual interest, erectile function, or depressed mood, with family members, friends, or even their own doctors. Because of that, many men may go undiagnosed and untreated. Physicians and their male patients need to establish a dialogue where topics of this nature can be freely discussed."

Professionals are predicting that in the near future, most men sixty-five or older will take testosterone, just as most menopausal women now take estrogen. To get to that point, though, certain steps need to be taken. The first is recognizing that andropause is a syndrome that can be treated. In a 1994 article in the *Journal of the American Medical Association*, Carl Heller and Gordon Myers say that andropause "is just as truly a syndrome based on endocrine disturbances as is the menopause syndrome in women."

---

96 Arver S, Dobs AS, Meikle AW, et al. "Improvement of sexual function in testosterone deficient men treated for one year with a permeation enhanced testosterone transdermal system." *J Urol* 155(5):1604–1608, 1996.

Identifying male menopause offers no threat to masculinity. Instead, it opens the doors to effective treatment and relief from the frustration of lowered testosterone that most men experience sooner or later in life. This is the first step.

Changing Perceptions

The next step to widespread testosterone therapy lies in changing the negative image of testosterone. Abuse of testosterone and other anabolic steroids (man-made, testosterone-like chemicals) by athletes and exaggerated reports of potential harm have constituted the bulk of press coverage of the subject. Although we do not promote the use of testosterone for bulking up or improving athletic performance, research shows that when monitored and administered in physiologic, non-abusive doses, natural testosterone has no negative side effects.

Other people are concerned that replacing testosterone will create a race of men who are bestially aggressive and hypersexual. The aim of all hormone replacement therapy is to replace only that which has been lost through the progression of time. Replacing testosterone to optimal levels only increases lost energy, boosts declining sex drive, and restores the physical and mental health a man experienced when he was younger. Testosterone therapy will not turn a peace-loving husband into the Wolfman.

Studies over the past decades show that replacing testosterone can help restore a man's health, although Dr. Dobs admits that, "Compared to estrogen research, we're fifteen years behind in investigating the benefits of testosterone." Some of the benefits of testosterone have been documented by Dr. Fran Kaiser, who runs a sexual dysfunction clinic at the St. Louis University School of Medicine. Dr. Kaiser has treated both hypogonadal young men and older men with low levels of testosterone. Her study on testosterone replacement in older men is one of the longest clinical trials of the hormone to date.

The Bone Building Hormone for Men

Even though osteoporosis is more often thought of as a problem that women face as they age, it is actually a serious concern for any elderly individual. In fact, one in eight men over age fifty will have an osteoporosis-related fracture. Tens of thousands of men suffer hip fractures every year, and a third of them die that same year. Unfortunately, the facts about osteoporosis in men are not widely understood.

Dr. Kaiser reported that older men with a testosterone deficiency were six times more likely to break a hip during a fall than younger men. By replacing this hormone to youthful levels, elderly men experience an increase in bone density, bone formation, and bone minerals, and an overall increase in energy. How and why testosterone can affect so much, we still don't know for certain. Dr. Kaiser says, "It appears as if testosterone is a major regulator, probably via a whole slew of other neurotransmitters, most of which we haven't yet identified."[97]

Energy to Spare

Dr. Kaiser's studies also indicated that men experienced an increase in overall physical energy when using testosterone. This may be due to testosterone's ability to increase the number of red

---

97 Kaiser F, Morley JE. "Gonadotropins, testosterone, and the aging male." *Neuro Aging* 15:559–563, 1994.

Marin P, Holmang S, Jonsson L, et al. "The effects of testosterone treatment on body composition and metabolism in middle-aged obese men." *Int J Obes* 16:991–997, 1992.

Marin P. "Testosterone and regional fat distribution." *Obesity Res* 3 Supp. 4:609S–612S, 1995.

blood cells, which provide the transport system for oxygen, taking it to all cells in the body. Oxygen is the fuel for every function that each cell, and therefore the body, performs. So the greater the number of red blood cells, the greater the amount of oxygen that can reach the body's cells. Red blood cell count should be monitored, however, because if it climbs too high, it can increase the risk of blood clots and stroke.

Muscle and Fat

These studies on testosterone prove that the hormone certainly controls more than just a man's sexual function. Professor Per Marin, of Goteborg, Sweden, performed two double-blind, placebo-controlled studies lasting about nine months, with the aim of raising serum testosterone to youthful levels. Marin and his associates found a significant decrease in body fat and a change in overall physical composition, most notably the disappearance of potbellies. This is due to decreasing triglyceride assimilation and improved use of existing fat. Another recent study of a small group of men taking the hormone indicated that it caused an increase in both muscle strength and in the diameter of muscle fibers. Supplementing the hormone also improved blood glucose levels, decreased blood pressure, and increased insulin sensitivity.[98]

Sexual Health

At the Endocrine Society meetings in Washington DC in June 1995, Dr. Fred Ellyin of the Chicago Medical School reported his findings: that as men age, they suffer a marked decrease in muscle

98 Marin P, Holmang S, Jonsson L, et al. "The effects of testosterone treatment on body composition and metabolism in middle-aged obese men." *Int J Obes* 16:991–997, 1992.

Marin P. "Testosterone and regional fat distribution." *Obesity Res* 3 Supp. 4:609–S612S, 1995.

strength, sexual performance, and male assertiveness, due to a drop in testosterone levels of more than 40 percent. His study of men from sixty to seventy-five years old who took low doses of testosterone weekly for two years showed that the hormone caused an increase in sexual desire and frequency of intercourse, as well as a marked improvement in the subjects' moods and outlooks on life. They also had lower cholesterol and body fat, with an increase in muscle strength.

Heart Health

Along with improving strength, energy, sexual function, and body composition, researchers are now discovering that testosterone also helps the heart stay healthy. Originally, too much serum testosterone was thought to be one of the major contributors to the high incidence of male heart disease. After all, since estrogen helped prevent heart disease in women, it was thought that testosterone must be the culprit. But researchers are beginning to realize that the sex hormones work differently in male and female bodies, and new studies show that the men who do have heart attacks tend to have low testosterone levels.

Dr. Gerald Phillips of Columbia University College of Physicians and Surgeons studied fifty-five men undergoing X-rays of their blood vessels. He found that lower testosterone levels accompanied higher incidence and severity of heart disease (determined by coronary clogging). Phillips also discovered that testosterone appears to raise the HDL cholesterol levels in the body. The boost in HDL was accompanied by a drop in LDL and overall cholesterol levels. This may be the primary reason for testosterone's preventative effect on heart disease.[99]

---

99 Phillips GB, Pinkernell BH, Jing TY. "The association of hypotestosteronemia with coronary artery disease in men." *Arterioscler Thromb* 614:701–706, 1994.

Brain Function

Testosterone also plays an important role in the functioning of the brain. In women, it is theorized that the great number of estrogen receptors in the brain can, at least partly, account for some of the emotional and thought attributes that are traditionally more prominent in women than in men. At the top of this list of female brain functions is an improved verbal fluency and verbal memory. In recent studies, it appears that testosterone does for the male brain what estrogen does for the female brain. As estrogen can influence a woman's mood, so can sufficient testosterone help a man experience less anxiety and irritability, and greater feelings of well-being. Testosterone also appears to have a profound impact on the way a man thinks and how well he performs learning and memory functions.

On June 14, 1996, a group of Johns Hopkins scientists led by Dr. Adrian Dobs presented the results of a study that researched testosterone's effect on the brain. Ten men with low levels of testosterone took a series of work, memory, coordination, and other learning tests when they were both on and off testosterone treatment. Results showed that testosterone supplementation improved results of the visual and spatial skills tests. The hormone also helped men have a better mental grasp of objects. These tests included fitting blocks into their correct spaces, identifying pictures, and remembering shapes and patterns. These are the skills that help a man work with three dimensional objects and read maps, two skills that are traditionally male.

On the other hand, when the subjects were not taking testosterone, their test results were lower in all of the categories. These men seemed to perform better on the verbal fluency and verbal memory tests. The verbal functions of our brain are the ones most influenced by the hormone estrogen. In some older men, testosterone levels drop so much that estrogen becomes the more prominent sex hormone, explaining the verbal test performance scores.

Dr. Kaiser and associates also performed a study using mice to test the relationship between testosterone and the brain functions of learning and memory. All the mice used had testosterone levels that were 70 percent lower than those of healthy, young mice, and half of them were given testosterone pellets. Researchers taught all the mice the path through a maze and then tested their retention one week later. The mice who received the testosterone learned the maze more quickly and remembered the path better than the placebo group.

No Evidence of Cancer at Physiologically Optimal Levels

One of the major concerns physicians have had with recommending widespread use of testosterone replacement is the fear that high levels of the hormone increase the chances of men developing prostate cancer. Some preliminary studies showed that testosterone produces dihydrotestosterone, which accelerates prostatic cancer growth. But two more recent studies indicate that giving low levels of the hormone does not increase dihydrotestosterone and does not increase the risk of prostate cancer.[100]

Young men have higher testosterone levels than older men, but prostate cancer is generally not found in young men. It stands to reason that testosterone cannot be the cause of prostate cancer. (However, once developed, prostate cancer's growth is exacerbated by testosterone.)

---

100 Carter HB, Pearson JD, Waclawiw Z, et al. "Prostate-specific antigen variability in men without prostate cancer: effect of sampling interval on prostate-specific antigen velocity." *Urology* 45(4):591–596, 1995.

Carter HB, Pearson JD, Metter EJ, et al. "Longitudinal evaluation of serum androgen levels in men with and without prostate cancer." *Prostate* 27(1):25–31, 1995.

A 1995 study by a Johns Hopkins research team headed by Dr. H. B. Carter examined three groups of age-matched men. The men in the first group were free of prostate cancer. In the second group, they had been diagnosed with benign prostate enlargement and had undergone a prostatectomy to remove it. The final group was diagnosed with current prostate cancer. The total testosterone and free testosterone levels for all the men were measured, showing no significant differences. The men who had been diagnosed with prostate cancer had no higher levels of testosterone than did the healthy men. Dr. Ellyin also reported that his study showed no rise in the test subjects' PSA levels and no enlargement of the prostate gland with testosterone treatment. These researchers concluded that high levels of testosterone do not increase the risk of prostate cancer.

The results of two more recent studies were reported at the 1996 International Congress of Endocrinology. A Baylor study indicated that eight men who took testosterone supplements for seventeen to eighty-six months showed no serious change in prostate specific antigen (PSA) levels or prostate size. Nor did PSA levels climb in the 122 men treated with testosterone for four years in a University of Utah study.[101]

The Patch

The University of Utah study was a part of the research used to determine the safety and effectiveness of a new form of testosterone treatment: a transdermal patch. Traditionally, the testosterone hormone could not be taken orally due to the deactivating role of the digestion process, so a synthetic testosterone was developed

---

101 Meikle AW, Arver S, Dobs AS, et al. "Pharmacokinetics and metabolism of a permeation-enhanced testosterone transdermal system in hypogonadal men: influence of application site—a clinical research center study." *J Clin Endocrinol Metab* 81(5):1832–1840, 1996.

that was made to be taken in tablet form. This method meant that the synthetic designer hormone had to pass through the digestive system, and reports showed that, in the long run, this was detrimental to liver function. The other option for treatment was injection which, aside from being both inconvenient and painful, was also the synthetically designed hormone. Also, injection treatment took place only once or twice a week.

In order to create a safer and more physiologic way to administer testosterone, several companies have developed transdermal patches or skin gels. Both of these methods use small amounts of natural testosterone, applied more frequently, which absorbs into the skin and then into the bloodstream. The patches are worn for a certain amount of time, during which the testosterone is slowly absorbed into the skin. Both of these methods eliminate the risk of liver problems, with the only consistent side effect reported by patch-users being some mild to moderate redness or itching at the site of the application.

Medical Supervision

Although with proper administration the fear of testosterone-induced prostate cancer may be unfounded, physicians still recommend that testosterone users regularly have their PSA levels checked. This is a wise procedure for any man who is entering middle- or old-age, whether or not he is using any hormone treatment. Cancer risk can be reduced even more when testosterone therapy is combined with other hormone treatments, including HGH and melatonin, which has been shown to retard the growth of prostate cancer. Even if cancer was not a concern, the potential for other side effects demands that an individual attempt to raise his testosterone to the optimal, safe level only under the supervision of a trained physician.

Some negative side effects include flushed or red skin, agitation, acne outbreak, increased dermal oil, irritability, and nervousness. Most of these side effects disappear when the dose of testosterone is reduced. With proper medical supervision, testosterone can be a beneficial and invaluable part of total hormone therapy.

TESTOSTERONE FOR WOMEN

Testosterone is not just for men. We have learned that replacing progesterone in women is just as important as replacing estrogen. We should not forget that testosterone, the quintessential male hormone, is also a female hormone. Unfortunately, we are even further behind in our research in female use of testosterone than we are in our understanding of male testosterone replacement.

Healthy women naturally have small amounts of testosterone in their bodies. In fact, it is produced by the female reproductive organs, the ovaries. As with estrogen and progesterone, a woman's testosterone levels drop as she ages. A woman could be diligently taking her estrogen and progesterone each day, and she may still not feel like herself. That is because she is ignoring another of her essential hormones: testosterone. If testosterone is not at its optimal level, the female body is still a bit out of balance. Since the goal is to truly replace all the hormones to a youthful level, testosterone must be included in the mix.

Increased Libido

The fact that women only have a small amount of testosterone in their bodies does not mean that the hormone is unimportant. Testosterone is important in triggering some of the processes a girl undergoes during puberty. Many researchers believe that one of testosterone's primary female functions is helping to control a woman's libido. Research also shows that testosterone levels, which fluctuate dramatically throughout the menstrual cycle, are highest just prior to ovulation. Combine this surge with the influx of progesterone, and it is no wonder that many women feel their greatest sexual drive and energy at this particular time.

Dr. Barbara Sherwin of McGill University in Montreal has studied testosterone replacement in post-menopausal women for the past twenty years. The most dramatic effect she has observed is how testosterone influences a woman's libido. With the decline in hormones at menopause, a woman's sex drive decreases. Some women lose interest in sex altogether. But Dr. Sherwin's studies showed that women who took the testosterone regained their desire for sex and enjoyed it more. These women frequently reported that they experienced more orgasms.[102]

Menopausal Relief

Testosterone does more for a woman than boost her libido. In fact, it appears that testosterone enhances the functions of estrogen. One of the primary uses of testosterone is for women who take estrogen and progesterone but still have no relief from severe menopausal symptoms. When these women begin taking testosterone as well, the mood swings and irritability disappear.

Bone Health

As discovered in tests with male testosterone supplementation, this hormone is also instrumental in strengthening the bones and preventing osteoporosis. We have seen that estrogen can slow the

102 Sherwin BB. "Affective changes with estrogen and androgen replacement therapy in surgically menopausal women." *J Affect Disord* 14(2):177–187, 1988.
Sherwin BB. "Estrogen and/or androgen replacement therapy and cognitive functioning in surgically menopausal women." *Psychoneuroendocrinology* 13(4):345–357, 1988.

destruction of bone, but not help rebuild it. Like progesterone, when testosterone is given with estrogen, the damaged bones begin to rebuild and strengthen. So rather than slowing the progression of osteoporosis, optimum hormone therapy can actually reverse it or even prevent it altogether.

Decreased Breast Cancer Risk

When women take testosterone in combination with their other hormones, their therapy is much more physiologic. This means that by adding testosterone to the mix, the body better accepts all the other hormones, with fewer side effects and increased benefits. One such benefit may be a decreased risk of breast cancer in women. Testosterone replacement is essential to a woman's overall physical and mental well-being.

What to Watch for

Because women naturally only have a very small amount of testosterone, it doesn't take a great deal to replace it to its physiologic levels. When women take only small doses of the hormone, there appear to be virtually no side effects. However, if the dose is too high, women can develop acne and unwanted hair growth on the body. Again, we are not trying to create super-human women; we only want to put back that which has been lost through the ravages of aging.

MELATONIN

Up to this point, all the hormones we have discussed in this chapter have been steroidal, or cholesterol-based hormones. Other hormones, including melatonin, HGH, thyroid, and thymus, are made up of a chain of amino acids. Each hormone has a specific sequence of amino acids which determines its function in the body.

Probably the most popular of these hormones is melatonin. It was the first hormone to make big news as an antiaging medicine and has been touted as the new super-substance that can do everything but walk the dog and wash the dinner dishes. You can buy melatonin supplements at almost any grocery store, and ads for the hormone still dot the pages of health food magazines. Part of this fervor was fueled by the publication of books such as *The Melatonin Miracle* by Walter Pierpaoli, MD, PhD, and William Regelson, MD, which outlines how melatonin helps keep us healthy.[103]

But this superhormone had a rather inauspicious beginning. Melatonin is manufactured and secreted by the pineal gland. This small organ was once considered a useless evolutionary remnant, like the appendix. In fact, melatonin itself was not discovered until 1958, when Dr. Lerner at Yale University isolated the molecule. Since then, we have learned much about this incredible substance. Scientists discovered that melatonin is made from the amino acid tryptophan, an essential amino acid. This means our bodies do not produce it. Instead, we must get tryptophan from the foods we eat. Tryptophan is found in meat and poultry, but the richest sources include dry-roasted sunflower seeds, pumpkin seeds, collard or turnip greens, and especially bananas and baked potatoes (with the skins). Once tryptophan is consumed, the body converts it into the neurotransmitter serotonin, which is involved in controlling mood. Then, at night, serotonin is converted into melatonin.

Widely Recommended Sleep Aid

Because of melatonin's nocturnal release, the initial clinical studies of the hormone focused on problems related to sleep and

103 Pierpaoli W, Regelson W. *The Melatonin Miracle.* New York: Simon and Schuster, 1995.

daily cycles. Researchers discovered that melatonin controls the natural rhythms, or circadian cycles, of the body, most notably the sleep-wake cycle.

In its capacity as a body clock, melatonin tells the body when to sleep and when to wake. It acts as a third eye, relying on the changing light to trigger its release. Light suppresses the release of melatonin, but when night falls, the dimming light, transferred through the eyes into the pineal gland, stimulates the release of more melatonin into the bloodstream. This is what causes us to feel sleepy. The levels peak at midnight and then gradually decrease throughout the rest of the night. In the morning, increasing light triggers melatonin production to decrease more rapidly and wake us up.

The changes in light are key to the secretion of melatonin. In fact, researchers discovered that blind people normally have no circadian rhythm of melatonin secretion and often suffer from sleep disorders. Sleep disorders are also common among the elderly. As with every other hormone, melatonin levels decline as we age. The lower levels mean that the sleep-wake cycle is not being regulated as well, so melatonin-deficient individuals are usually not getting the sleep they need. These people not only toss and turn all night but have difficulty functioning well during the day. They are fatigued and have trouble concentrating. Any of us who have spent sleepless nights know how hard the morning after can be.

So researchers set out to determine if the cyclical release of melatonin indicated that it could be used as a sleep aid and provide help for insomniacs and the elderly. What they found was that by lowering the core body temperature, melatonin increases the body's ability to relax and sleep. In the case of insomnia, melatonin supplementation was found to increase the test subjects' total sleep time and improve their daytime alertness. Melatonin also reduces the time needed to fall asleep, promotes more vivid dreaming, reduces the number of times subjects awaken during the night, and stimulates a greater quality of sleep, or a greater amount of deep, REM sleep.

A 1995 study showed that evening doses of melatonin did, in fact, stimulate sleep. It did not delay or suppress REM sleep, and did not induce the hangover effects that are common with other over-the-counter drug sleep aids. The same research team also tested the effects of nighttime levels of melatonin given during the day. All of the test subjects indicated that the hormone increased sleep duration, daytime sleepiness, and fatigue. These studies show that although the light cycle is what triggers the release of melatonin, the hormone can stimulate sleep at any time of day.[104]

Melatonin also secretes different amounts depending on body temperature. Research has shown that the amount of melatonin in the blood increases when warm bath water is heated by as little as 2 degrees centigrade. For this reason, a hot bath taken in the evening can help you fall asleep faster. Interestingly, if the water is lukewarm, the amount of melatonin does not increase. It takes hot water to stimulate the conarium in our brain so that melatonin is secreted.

Of course, melatonin is only one of many sleep aid options people can choose from when they go to the store. But it appears to be by far the most natural choice, and therefore the least likely to cause side effects. Many of the drugs that stimulate sleep will also suppress the dream, or REM state of sleep, which is considered the most physically beneficial time during sleep. These drugs also

104 Dollins AB, Zhdanova IV, Wurtman RJ, et al. "Effect of inducing nocturnal serum melatonin concentrations in daytime on sleep, mood, body temperature, and performance." *Proc Natl Acad Sci USA* 91:1824–1828, 1994.
Zhdanova IV, Wurtman RJ, Lynch HJ, et al. "Sleep-inducing effects of low doses of melatonin ingested in the evening." *Clin Pharmacol Ther* 57:552–558, 1995.

tend to lose their effect over time and can be addictive. And at high doses, sleeping pills can be lethal. Melatonin, on the other hand, doesn't have any of these negative drawbacks.

Jet Lag Treatment

Because of this power, melatonin has also been used to treat jet lag, the fatigue and disorientation that travelers experience as their bodies try to adjust to a new time zone and a new light and dark cycle. A study published in the *British Medical Journal* in 1994 showed that taking melatonin helped travelers sleep and reduced their fatigue and disorientation. Users also reported a greater ability to focus and fewer mood swings.

HGH Booster

As great as these benefits may be, melatonin does a lot more than just regulate our sleep-wake cycles. In fact, it appears that this one hormone helps regulate the functioning of our entire body. Many of the functions of melatonin may sound like some of these we've discussed in relation to HGH. This is because melatonin regulates, or at least influences, the release of HGH from the pituitary gland. Some of melatonin's benefits could well be attributed to the work that HGH does in the body.

The relationship between melatonin and HGH is strong. Melatonin tells our bodies to sleep, and it is throughout REM sleep that HGH is released. During puberty, melatonin levels fall, telling our brain to trigger the physical and sexual changes that need to occur at that time. Interestingly, that is the time the body's natural production and secretion of HGH begins to decline, so some researchers believe the secretion of melatonin is directly proportional to how much HGH we have in our bodies. However, more recent studies indicate that optimal levels of melatonin cannot entirely bring the levels of HGH up to where they need to be for maximum health, particularly in elderly individuals.

Antiaging Benefits

Not only does melatonin influence and sometimes regulate HGH, it also has a strong effect on the other hormones and the entire body. The pineal gland uses melatonin to communicate with all the body's cells. This hormone has the unique ability not only to affect hormone receptors on the outside of the cell, but also to enter the cell and communicate directly with the cell's DNA in order to get the cell or the organ to behave a certain way.

Around age forty-five, the pineal gland seems to become run down. Melatonin secretion slowly declines for years, but at middle age, the hormone levels plummet. This phenomenon then triggers the other hormone levels to decline. It doesn't happen overnight, but slowly, one by one, hormone levels in our body drop. Consequently, the functioning of our body systems also slows down, and we experience what is known as aging.

Long before telomeres and telomerase were touted as parts of the biological aging clock, this unique function of the pineal gland had already earned it the name of the aging clock. It is as if, by reducing the flow of melatonin, this gland is informing the body of its age and saying, "It's quitting time." To test this theory, Drs. Walter Pierpaoli and William Regelson, pioneers in hormone therapy, traded the pineal glands of four-month-old mice (approximately teenagers in human terms) with those of Twenty-four-month-old mice (equal to sixty-five- to seventy-year-old humans). The young mice with the old pineal glands began to age very rapidly. This was evident in physical features (deteriorated hair and skin quality), as well as in the decreased energy and vitality the mice exhibited. These young mice also died 30 percent earlier than the control mice. Even though these young mice were in good health at the time the study began, the old pineal gland told the body that it was time to age, and the organs responded by shutting down.

This discovery opened the door for all that we know about hormones and their antiaging benefits. If the decrease in melatonin is responsible for aging the body, then theoretically we could stop aging by simply raising the hormone back to healthy levels. We could reset the aging clock. Finally, with this realization, aging was no longer an inevitable physical condition. It was a disease that could be stopped.

The theory that melatonin supplementation could rejuvenate the body and fight the disease of aging was also tested in the Pierpaoli and Regelson study. Not only did they observe that the old pineal gland induced rapid aging in young mice, but young pineal glands restored youth to old mice. The old mice suddenly had improved fur, greater energy, and behaved like young mice. Researchers also proved that the pineal transplant helped restore the shrunken thymus gland to its original size in the old mice. Since the thymus gland is one of the key organs of the immune system, the mice were then better able to fight off the diseases of old age. At one point in the study, the doctors reported that just from looking at the mice, they had difficulty telling which ones were four months old and which were twenty-four months old.

Finally came the true test of the power of the pineal gland. Not only did a young pineal gland improve the health of these mice, it actually extended their lives. Old mice with a young pineal gland lived 30 percent longer than normal, and researchers say they were youthful until their deaths.[105]

---

105 Pierpaoli W, Regelson W. "Pineal control of aging: effect of melatonin and pineal grafting on aging mice." *Proc Natl Acad Sci USA* 94:787–791, 1994.

Resetting the aging clock allows us to slow down, and even reverse, physical aging. The increase in melatonin levels can trick the body into thinking it is time to be young, and not time to shut down. The youthful message the body receives affects almost all of our body systems.

Sexual Rejuvenation

One of these affected body systems is the reproductive system. People who take melatonin report a dramatic increase in sexual drive and energy. This sexual rejuvenation is partly due to the overall energy increase that comes with higher levels of melatonin. But Dr. Pierpaoli proved that the hormone had a direct influence on the sex organs themselves. As mammals age, ovaries and testes tend to shrink, generally because of decreased levels of the sex hormones. Melatonin therapy may be able to regenerate these organs and improve sexual function.

Dr. Pierpaoli gave melatonin to aging mice between seven and eight years old. These mice, both male and female, had reproductive organs that showed none of the shrinkage seen in other elderly mice. In fact, both the ovaries and the testes were twice the size of those in the control group and looked like the reproductive organs of younger mice. This study proved that melatonin could stimulate the production of sex hormones, which regenerated the reproductive organs and increased the sexual behavior in mice.[106]

Heart Health

Melatonin also plays an important role in maintaining heart health. Melatonin stimulates the release of HGH, which builds

---

106 Pierpaoli W, Bulian D, Dall'Ara A, et all. "Circadian melatonin and young-to-old pineal grafting postpone aging and maintain juvenile conditions of reproductive functions in mice and rats." *Exp Gerontol* 32(4–5):587–602, 1997.

the muscles of the heart, making it less susceptible to heart disease. Melatonin is also important in regulating cholesterol levels and blood pressure, both of which rise as we age, increasing our risk of stroke and heart attack. Humans who have high cholesterol are generally deficient in melatonin. In animals, removing the pineal gland causes the cholesterol and triglyceride levels to rise dramatically. Melatonin also appears to help maintain healthy triglyceride and cholesterol levels, even in an unhealthy, high-cholesterol diet.

Immune System Booster

One of melatonin's greatest powers is its ability to boost the immune system. The Pierpaoli-Regelson study mentioned earlier indicated that a young pineal gland, secreting greater amounts of melatonin, was able to restore the thymus to its healthy size. The thymus is the gland responsible for the production of T-cells, which fight off infectious organisms and cancerous cells. After childhood, the thymus begins to shrink until, by age eighty, it is almost impossible to find. When the thymus shrinks, the production of T-cells declines, leaving the body's defenses weakened and susceptible to the invasion of bacteria and viruses. By restoring the thymus gland to its youthful size, melatonin increases the number of T-cells available to fight off invading organisms.

As melatonin roams the body, it stimulates the production of more antibodies and helps fight off viral infections. Another study published in the November/December 1994 issue of *Psychosomatic Medicine* reported that a melatonin deficiency can severely weaken our immune system. Physicians at the San Diego Veterans Affairs Medical Center studied the effects of sleep deprivation of twenty-three healthy men between the ages of twenty-two and sixty-one. When the men were denied sleep between 3:00 a.m. and 7:00 a.m., their melatonin levels were lower than normal. More interestingly, these same men also had substantially reduced white blood cell activity, particularly the natural killer (NK) cells. These are the cells that are most vital in protecting the body from viruses and cancer.[107]

Possible Cancer Prevention

These studies suggest that melatonin could be a powerful anti-cancer treatment. In particular, breast cancer may prove to respond well to melatonin therapy. Since one in nine women will develop breast cancer at some time in her life, the possibility that melatonin may be an effective preventative treatment is exciting. Studies have shown that women with low levels of melatonin are at greater risk for developing breast cancer. When the cancer does appear, the pineal gland starts pumping out greater amounts of melatonin to go to work fighting the invaders. In this way, melatonin not only influences the immune system but acts as part of it. Ironically and unfortunately, traditional cancer treatments like chemotherapy suppress the secretion of melatonin.[108]

A study in the *British Journal of Cancer* in June 1993 reported that combining melatonin with the immune-boosting protein interleukin-2 was at least partially effective in treating cancer of the digestive tract in terminally ill patients.[109]

---

107 Irwin M, Mascovich A, Gillin JC, et al. "Partial sleep deprivation reduces natural killer cell activity in humans." *Psychosom* Med 56(6):493–498, 1994.

108 Lissoni P, Barni S, Meregalli S, et al. "Modulation of cancer endocrine therapy by melatonin: a phase II study of tamoxifen plus melatonin in metastatic breast cancer patients progressing under tamoxifen alone." *Br J Cancer* 71:854–856, 1995.

109 Lissoni P, Barni S, Tancini G, et al. "Immunotherapy with subcutaneous low-dose Interleukin-2 and the pineal indole melatonin as a new effective therapy in advanced cancers of the digestive tract." *Br J Cancer* 67(6):1404–1407, 1993.

These cancers, including pancreatic, stomach, liver, and colon cancer, do not respond well to chemotherapy and are often considered untreatable. Of those who received the melatonin treatment, 23 percent responded positively, and in 31 percent of the cases, the disease was stabilized. The numbers may not look all that impressive until you consider the fact that these patients had basically been given up for dead by the medical community. In this case, a 23 percent improvement rate can be considered a medical breakthrough! In the future, it may be possible to combine melatonin with other promising anti-cancer treatments to produce an even greater cure rate.

Antioxidant Properties

This cancer-fighting power comes from the fact that melatonin is, in reality, a powerful antioxidant. Antioxidants are the body's defense against free radicals, the molecules that spread cancerous growth by attacking our cells. In fact, melatonin appears to be a more powerful antioxidant than even vitamins C and E. Free radicals most often target the cell membrane and the cell's DNA, completely altering the structure of the cell. Melatonin has an advantage over other antioxidants in protecting the cells. Not only does melatonin neutralize free radicals that attack the protective membranes of our cells, but by getting into the nucleus, melatonin is able to directly protect the DNA inside, as well.

Dr. Russell Reiter, from the University of Texas Health Science Center in San Antonio, showed the protection melatonin can offer by being able to freely enter and permeate all parts of a cell. To prove this point, Reiter used a cancer-promoting agent called safrole which, when given alone, quickly oxidizes the liver cells and destroys the DNA. Before giving test mice safrole shots, Reiter gave them tiny doses of melatonin. The melatonin was able to enter the cells and directly protect the DNA from the free radical damage. The group of mice who received small doses of melatonin showed 41 percent less damage than their counterparts who received none of the hormone. With another group of mice, Reiter raised the dose of melatonin slightly, resulting in only 1% as much liver damage as the control mice.

Protection from Poisons

More recently, Reiter has shown that melatonin can also protect from the damage caused by radiation, and that it can safeguard mice from the effects of a deadly herbicide. Reiter also believes that melatonin may be instrumental in preventing cataracts, which are caused by the oxidation that occurs on the lenses of the eyes.[110]

Best Supervised by Your Doctor

With all of these amazing benefits, it is no wonder melatonin is such a popular supplement. It also appears to be safe. In studies using varying doses of melatonin, the only reported side effects included high-dose-induced headaches, nausea, chronic grogginess, and nightmares. Despite the apparent safety, self-prescribed melatonin users still experience some problems.

One of the main problems lies with the over-the-counter varieties of the supplement. Because melatonin is not a regulated substance, almost anyone can manufacture it. Some formulations may be poor quality and not completely pure. This increases your risk of experiencing the side effects mentioned above, and some people have reported another problem: that the effect of melatonin wears off suddenly. Melatonin stimulates the release of several of

---

110 Reiter RJ, Tan DX, Poeggeler B, et al. "Melatonin as a free radical scavenger: implications for aging and age-related diseases." *Ann NY Acad Sci* 719:1–12, 1994.

the other hormones in the body, including HGH and the sex hormones. This can be of great benefit, but it also increases the need for physician monitoring. If your aim is youthful balance, remember, too much of any hormone throws off your body's functioning as much as too little.

THYROID HORMONE

The thyroid is another hormone that is essential to maintaining a healthy balance in the body. There are two types of thyroid hormones: thyroxine (T4) and triiodothyronine (T3). T4 is inactive and kept in reserve, while T3 is the active hormone. T4 is converted into T3 when the body needs thyroid hormone. Thyroid hormone controls the temperature of the body, and through temperature it controls growth, differentiation, and metabolism of each cell in the body, most notably those in the brain. It also controls how fast we use the fuel that we consume, particularly carbohydrates and fat. This, in turn, helps to regulate our temperature and body fat percentage. Thyroid also encourages the manufacture of glucose, which helps fuel the body. Additionally, these hormones stimulate the production of key proteins that form the building blocks of our body's cells. By controlling these aspects of the body's metabolism, thyroid also gives us energy.

The thyroid hormones are produced in the thyroid gland, which is located in the lower part of the neck and made of two connected lobes that look something like a butterfly or shield. In fact, the name *thyroid* comes from a Greek word meaning "shield." This gland uses iodine to produce the various thyroid hormones. We get the needed iodine from the food we eat. Some areas, including the Great Lakes region of the United States, are naturally iodine deficient, so iodine must be added to certain foods like salt and bread in order to give the body sufficient amounts to produce thyroid hormone.

The release of thyroid hormone is controlled by thyroid-stimulating hormone (TSH), which is produced in the pituitary gland. Low circulating levels of thyroid hormone are detected by the hypothalamus, which then tells the pituitary to release TSH. In high enough amounts, this hormone prompts the thyroid gland to produce and secrete more of the thyroid hormones. Then, when sufficient thyroid is detected in the blood, the hypothalamus communicates with the pituitary to stop or slow the production of TSH. In this way, the hormone levels are kept balanced in a healthy body.

Because of this feedback loop, very high levels of TSH in the blood indicate a hormonal imbalance and a problem in the body. Lots of circulating TSH often means that the pituitary is trying hard to stimulate the release of thyroid hormones, but the thyroid gland is not responding sufficiently. This condition is known as *thyroid origin hypothyroidism*. Hypothyroidism occurs when, for a number of reasons, the thyroid produces too little of the necessary hormones.

Some researchers estimate that this condition affects approximately 3 percent to 5 percent of the population, while others believe the number is closer to 40 percent. It also seems to be more common in women and the elderly. At least 8 percent of all women will have a thyroid dysfunction after pregnancy. In the older age group, the pituitary slows down the production of TSH, which then also reduces thyroid hormone production. This is known as *pituitary origin hypothyroidism* and is seen frequently in our practice.

There is another type of hypothyroidism that results from the inability to convert T4 to biologically active T3. Blood levels of TSH and T4 are normal, but the patient is still suffering from hypothyroid symptoms. The diagnosis can only be made if free T3 is measured.

Symptoms of Hypothyroidism

Hypothyroidism may not be accompanied by any symptoms, and when symptoms do exist, they will vary according to the degree of hormone deficiency. The most common symptoms include:

- Fatigue that is most pronounced in the mornings and afternoons.
- Lower than normal body temperature. A body temperature that is consistently below 97.6° F is a strong indication of hypothyroidism. Sufferers complain of feeling cold all the time, particularly in the hands and feet.
- A greater susceptibility to colds and other viruses. Hypothyroid patients generally show a weakened immune system.
- Depression and mood swings are also common symptoms of hypothyroidism. In fact, some researchers believe that postpartum depression may be due, at least in part, to the thyroid imbalance women experience after giving birth.

Based on the preceding list, you can see that many of the symptoms of hypothyroidism are often also related to the normal progression of age, and can therefore be easily overlooked and untreated. The following is a list of other signs of hypothyroidism:

- weakness
- cramping
- weight gain
- tingling in the fingers
- dry skin
- constipation
- joint pain or arthritis

- slowed heart rate
- headaches
- high cholesterol
- memory impairment and inability to concentrate
- infertility or menstrual irregularity in women

Home Test for Hypothyroidism

If you have a number of these symptoms, you may have a mild to severe case of hypothyroidism. If you are over age fifty or female, your chances are even greater. But as you can imagine, many of these symptoms may also be indications of other illnesses and not necessarily indicative of an underactive thyroid. So before you rush out to your doctor and demand a multitude of thyroid hormone levels tests, take a simple home test first.

Dr. Broda Barnes, who spent most of his life studying the thyroid gland and its hormones, developed a simple test for determining your basal body temperature. Your body temperature is important because it is a direct measure of your body's metabolic rate which, as explained above, is controlled by the thyroid. Dr. Barnes recommends testing for your basal temperature before getting out of bed in the morning. When you wake up, put a shaken-down thermometer in your armpit for ten minutes. If the temperature reading is below 97.2° F for several days in a row, Dr. Barnes believes it is a strong indication of hypothyroidism.[111]

In our clinical experience at the Palm Springs Life Extension Institute, we have found that taking your temperature orally for three minutes, while at rest during the afternoon, is a good way of assessing thyroid status. A temperature below 98° F is a good indication of hypothyroidism.

---

111 Barnes B. *Hypothyroidism: The Unsuspected Illness*. New York: Harper Collins, 1976.

Treatment Brings Back Energy

The only treatment for hypothyroidism is thyroid hormone replacement, which has been rather common for years, using T4 and T3 combinations. The patients who take the hormone say that, more than anything, they just feel better and have a lot more energy.

Let us explain how thyroid can act as an energizer. We need adequate energy for everything we do, beginning at the cellular level. The mitochondria (tiny cellular components) are responsible for burning the oxygen that we breathe and turning it into adenosine triphosphate (ATP), the substance which fuels the entire body. So what fuels the vital mitochondria? Thyroid. If there is not enough thyroid hormone, specifically T3, then the mitochondria cannot do their job as effectively, and less ATP is produced. You experience the hormone deficiency as an overall lack of energy.

Influencing the Brain

Thyroid's cellular energizing ability also has a significant influence on the functioning of the brain. In fact, infants with an underactive thyroid almost always develop learning disabilities and often suffer more serious mental retardation. Patients taking thyroid hormone report being able to think quicker and more clearly, and remember better. They also report improved mood, fewer mood swings, and less depression. In fact, in his book *The Superhormone Promise*, Dr. William Regelson says that he believes the most common forms of depression could be easily and safely treated by restoring physiologic levels of thyroid.[112]

---

112 Regelson W, Coleman C. *The Superhormone Promise*. New York: Simon and Schuster, 1996.

Supplemental Treatment for Diabetes

Thyroid hormone replacement may also be a supplemental treatment for diabetes. The thyroid hormone controls metabolism, and diabetes is a metabolic disorder. Also, thyroid hormone is closely involved in the production of glucose, and sufficient levels of thyroid hormone may help normalize blood-sugar levels.

Research Reports on Cancer

Some research also reports that thyroid hormone may be able to reverse certain types of cancer. The research in both of these fields is still very young, but we will learn even more about the benefits of thyroid hormone replacement as studies continue.

Links Between Thyroid and Heart Health

Concrete results are now available to document the link between thyroid and heart health. Researchers from Cornell University Medical College report that thyroid hormone is important to the health of the heart muscle and circulatory system. In their study, thyroid replacement yielded a quick improvement in cardiac output and cardiac contractility, and a decrease in vascular resistance. On the other hand, untreated hypothyroidism can lead to an enlarged heart (cardiomyopathy), and worsening heart failure. In severe cases, lack of treatment may cause the sufferer to lapse into a coma. Fortunately, this extreme is rare.[113]

Another study from the Oklahoma Transplantation Institute showed that thyroid treatment increased the success of heart transplants. Seventy recipients were treated with the hormone,

---

113 Althaus BU, Staub JJ, Ryff-De Leche A, et al. "LDL/MDL changes in subclinical hypothyroidism: possible risk factors for coronary heart disease." *Clin Endocrinol.* 28: 157–163, 1988.

Klein I. "Thyroid hormone and the cardiovascular system." *Am J Med* 88(6):631–637, 1990.

and all but three of the patients showed immediate healthy post-transplant heart function. In the other three patients, cardiac function became normal after a maximum of twenty-four hours of mechanical support.[114]

Immune System Protection

Thyroid may also aid in transplant success by improving the body's immune function. Sufficient release of thyroid hormone stimulates the formation of lymphocytes, the cells that attack viruses, bacteria, fungi, and other invading substances. Thyroid also promotes the production in the liver of phagocytes, a type of white blood cell that roams the body attacking invaders before they can do any harm.

Dr. Max Laurie of the University of Pennsylvania tested just how much thyroid can influence the immune system when he infected groups from two different breeds of rabbit with a highly contagious strain of tuberculosis bacteria. As expected, one group of rabbits developed the full-blown disease, and the other breed, infected with the same amount of TB bacteria as the first group, did not. Laurie explained that the first group of rabbits, as a breed, had very low levels of thyroid. The disease-free group, however, naturally produced higher-than-normal levels of thyroid hormone. The disease-fighting hormones produced by the thyroid kept these rabbits healthy.[115]

114 Novitzky D, Cooper DK, Chaffin JS, et al. "Improved cardiac allograft function following triiodothyronine therapy to both donor and recipient." *Transplantation* 49(2):311–316, 1990.

115 Laurie MB. *Resistance to Tuberculosis: Experimental Studies in Native and Acquired Defensive Mechanisms*. Cambridge, MA: Harvard University Press, 1964.

Under Watchful Eyes

Studies show that thyroid hormone treatment is safe and produces no allergic reactions. But as with all of the hormones, thyroid replacement must be carefully monitored by a qualified physician. Too much thyroid is just as dangerous as too little. If you take too much of the hormone, you may start to experience symptoms of hyperthyroidism. This includes feeling warm all the time, hyperactivity, a sense of nervousness, rapid heart beat, tremor, irritability, and insomnia. In cases of severe excess, or years of mild thyroid excess, the hormone could cause a serious heart rhythm problem and increase the risk of heart attack. Some studies also show that too much thyroid will rob your body of calcium, thereby increasing the risk of osteoporosis.

Since thyroid secretion is also controlled by the pituitary gland, other hormones can influence how the thyroid hormone works. For example, HGH can stimulate the body's production of thyroid hormone. Some studies have shown that HGH treatment may even be able to normalize thyroid function. Because of the way the hormones work synergistically, your levels of thyroid should be supervised as closely as all the other hormones in the body as part of a total hormone gene therapy program.[116]

THYMIC HORMONES

The thymus gland is located behind the sternum, or chest bone. It is very large at birth and disappears by the time you are forty or fifty. It is vital in providing immunity to the body. No matter how healthy and strong the heart, muscles, and other systems are, if the immune system isn't functioning properly, a common cold

---

116 Fraser WD, Biggart EM, O'Reilly DJ, et al. "Are biochemical tests of thyroid function of any value in monitoring patients receiving thyroxine replacement?" *Br Med J* 293:808–810, 1986.

can be deadly. As we age, our immune functions slow down and are not nearly as effective at fighting off diseases as they once were. As a result, bacteria and viruses lodge themselves in our systems and slowly kill us. In the human species, the thymus gland is genetically programmed to totally atrophy by the end of your forties. No wonder most cancers occur after this age.

Immune System Booster

Medical professionals have long known that the thymus gland is essential to the health of the immune system. Only recently, however, have physicians begun trying to rejuvenate the immune system by prescribing thymic hormones or peptides. What they've found is impressive. Thymus is the peptide of tomorrow; it is on the horizon and poised to become a "super-hormone." Don't be too surprised if, within a few short years, the articles and advertisements extolling the virtues of thymic supplements are as abundant as those for DHEA or melatonin.

We've already briefly addressed the role of the thymus in our discussions of HGH and melatonin. The function of the thymus gland is to nurture T-lymphocytes (T-cells), the white blood cells that fight viral infections and cancerous cells. To become mature, all T-cells must reside in the thymus gland for a period of time. During this time, they become either CD4 cells or CD8 cells. The CD4 cells are known as *helper cells* because they help the immune system by recognizing foreign substances on contact. CD8 cells are called *T-suppressor/cytotoxic*, or *killer cells*, and destroy the invaders once they have been identified by the CD4 cells. Once the T-cells have matured and differentiated into CD4 or CD8 cells, they are released into the body. Through these functions, the thymus gland basically controls the immune system.

The thymus gland has an interesting tendency to shrink as we age. This shrinking actually begins in our teens and twenties. By age forty, most of the thymic gland has been replaced by fat, and both the cortex and medulla have become severely atrophied. By age eighty, the thymus gland has all but disappeared. For many years, this shrinking was ignored by the medical world, since it was viewed as a normal and inevitable part of aging.

But some physicians realized that if the thymus gland controls the immune system, and decreased immunity comes with old age, then restoring the thymus might help people resist disease well into old age.

One of these physicians is Dr. Carson B. Burgstiner. Dr. Burgstiner first became aware of thymic peptides and their ability to fight disease when he contracted hepatitis B while operating on an infected patient. After several years of treatment, he was still a carrier for the disease. This frustration prompted him to seek alternative treatments. He began taking a thymic peptide and vitamin complex purchased at a health food store, and within six weeks he was no longer a carrier of hepatitis.[117]

With this personal discovery, Dr. Burgstiner and several colleagues began treating themselves and their patients with thymic peptide. One of the first studies showed that the thymic formula increased the serum levels of thymosin, one of the many thymic peptides present in extracts of the thymus gland, by 100 percent. A derivative called thymosin-alpha 1 has been shown to stimulate T-lymphocyte activity, slightly improving immune function.[118]

---

117 Burgstiner CB. "Cure for hepatitis? 'Physician, heal thyself,' and he did." *J Med Assoc Ga* 80(1):21–22, 1991.

118 Eckert K, et al. "Thymosin-alpha 1 effects, in vitro, on lymphokine-activated killer cells from patients with primary immunodeficiencies: preliminary results." *Int J Immunopharmacology* 16(12):1019–1025, 1994.

Three years after treating his patients with thymic formula, Dr. Burgstiner reported amazing results. Eighty-four cases of hepatitis B were completely arrested, as were thirty-two cases of hepatitis C. Twenty-eight of his patients with rheumatoid arthritis found that they no longer needed to rely on their traditional treatments with prednisone, methotrexate, or gold shots. With thymic formula treatment, twelve patients with systemic lupus were found to be asymptomatic, and ten cases of multiple sclerosis, twelve of psoriasis, and seven of skin inflammation were arrested. Burgstiner also reported that three patients scheduled to have liver transplants no longer needed them, having recovered from their hepatitis with the help of thymic hormone treatment. The treatment also helped liver and heart transplant patients who contracted hepatitis B through blood transfusions.

In another recent study, thirty-three patients infected with the hepatitis B virus were randomly assigned to receive the thymic peptide thymosin, or another treatment called interferon alpha (INF-alpha). At six months, both groups showed improvement, but after six additional months of monitoring, those who had received the thymosin had a 41.2 percent complete response compared to 25 percent improvement in the INF-alpha group. Researchers concluded that thymosin was not only able to promote disease remission but sustain it as well. It was also well tolerated by all the test subjects.[119]

Dr. Burgstiner points out that not only are these numbers impressive, but so is the minimal time it took to see the effects of treatment. These dramatic results were often evident within three months, and in the case of hepatitis B, the virus was arrested

119 Andreone P, Cursaro C, Gramenzi A, et al. "A randomized controlled trial of thymosin-alpha 1 versus interferon alpha treatment in patients with hepatitis B e antigen antibody—and hepatitis B virus DNA—positive chronic hepatitis B." *Heptatology* 24(4):774–777, 1996.

in only six weeks. In the United States, there are three hundred thousand new cases of hepatitis B reported each year, and 1.5 million hepatitis-related deaths annually. With these numbers, the indications for thymic treatment are great indeed.

Adjunct Treatment for AIDS

It also appears that thymic peptides could be used to help treat another prominent killer: AIDS. The connection between the function of the thymus and the development of AIDS is not difficult to see. The immune deficiency seen in AIDS is similar to that seen in children with rare thymus disorders, and French studies have shown that patients with advanced HIV infection have low levels of some thymic peptides. The thymus is responsible for maturing T-cells, while the HIV virus destroys them, bringing on AIDS. This makes the sufferer susceptible to all kinds of infection and disease. So by stimulating the production of T-cells, thymic formulas could likely slow the reproduction of the HIV virus, or at least prevent HIV infection from converting to AIDS.

The February 1993 issue of *AIDS Treatment News* reported a study by Dr. Marcus Conant of San Francisco. This double-blind, forty-eight-week study involved 354 asymptomatic HIV-infected patients. All of the volunteers took AZT, and approximately half were also given thymopentin, another thymic peptide, while the other half took a placebo.

At the end of the study, fourteen of the volunteers who took the placebo developed AIDS symptoms, as compared to only four in the group who took the thymopentin.[120]

---

120 Conant MA, Calabrese LH, Thompson SE, et al. "Maintenance of CD4+ cells by thymopentin in asymptomatic HIV-infected subjects: results of a double-blind, placebo-controlled study." *AIDS* 6(11):1335–1339, 1992.

Endocrine, Nervous, and Cardiovascular System Connections

The results of other trials concerning thymic peptides and AIDS are still coming in, as are reports of how these peptides affect other diseases and other body systems. For example, the congenital absence of the thymus gland is associated with unhealthy alterations of the pituitary gland, adrenal gland, thyroid, and ovaries. Another early pioneer in thymus gland research, Dr. Walter Pierpaoli, was among the first to identify the dependency of the central nervous system's development on the thymus gland, primarily that the thymus is important to the development of the brain cells. As a result, the age-related deterioration of learning and memory abilities has also been linked to the atrophy of the thymus gland. Another physician from the University of Miami discovered that the buildup of plaque in the blood vessel walls is a result of immune system failure, and therefore, thymic failure.

These connections suggest that thymic peptide replacement could improve the health of the endocrine, central nervous, and cardiovascular systems.

Thymic Peptides and Lupus

Dr. Burgstiner also reported that in his treatment with thymic fractions, lupus cases were arrested. Another study, published in the February 1995 issue of *Lupus*, reported a definite link between thymic peptides and the disease. Fourteen women and two men between the ages of eleven and sixty-six all developed systemic lupus erythematosus after having had their thymus glands surgically removed. Half of the study group developed the disease within only three years. Most commonly, patients experienced polyarthritis, or arthritis in more than one joint, occurring in fifteen of the sixteen patients. Other common symptoms were skin rashes and fever. Most significantly, thymic activity in these patients was basically undetectable compared with normal controls.[121]

Herpes Studies

Thymic peptides or fractions have also been tested to determine their effectiveness in treating recurring viral infections like herpes simplex and papilloma (viral benign tumor of the larynx). These infections are difficult to treat with traditional antiviral therapy, but a compromised cellular immunity does seem to play a role in the development of the diseases. One 1994 study concluded that the thymic fraction, thymopentin, could be an effective treatment for these viral infections. And unlike the traditional antiviral drugs, thymopentin's effect is long-lasting, with benefits continuing after the treatment is discontinued.[122]

Improving Quality of Life for Cancer Patients

Thymic peptides also show promise for treating cancer patients. In some studies, the levels of thymulin, another thymic fraction, have been found to be much lower among cancer patients than in healthy individuals the same age. We also know that thymic peptides can stimulate the immune system and mobilize lymphocytes and T-cells.

For example, one study tested the effect of thymopentin on postoperative infection among two hundred sixty cancer patients. The treatment prevented a drop in the CD3- and CD4-positive T-cell levels among elderly cancer patients who underwent surgery.

---

121 Mevorach D, Perrot S, Buchanan NM, et al. "Appearance of systemic lupus erythematosus after thymectomy: four case reports and review of the literature." *Lupus* 4(1):33–37, 1995.

122 Sundal E, Bertelletti D. "Management of viral infections with thymopentin." *Arzneimittel-Forschung* 44(7):866–871, 1994.

The treatment group also had a lower incidence of postoperative infection than did the control group. Among those in the study who did develop an infection, it was far less severe among patients who were treated with thymopentin.[123]

Thymic Peptides and Wasting Syndrome

In 1964, it was demonstrated that peptides from the thymic tissue could prevent many of the manifestations of wasting syndrome caused by thymectomy. One technique used to discover the importance of the function of the thymus was to remove it from young animals and study the resultant changes. When the thymus gland is removed in small animals, the animals experience profound wasting.[124]

This wasting syndrome is characterized by an increased incidence of infection and cancer (immune suppression), failure to grow, allergies, neuromuscular weakness, and autoimmune diseases (immune dysfunction). Greater susceptibility to infection and cancer has also been shown to be directly attributable to the dramatic decrease in peripheral white blood cells called lymphocytes. While rearing the thymectomized animal in a sterile environment prevented the increased incidence of infection, it did not eliminate all the symptoms caused by removal of the thymus gland.

This research suggested that the thymus gland produces substances that are important in the development and maintenance of the immune system. Although the relationship of this observation to the wasting syndrome was not clearly

123 Braga M, Costantini E, Di Francesco A, et al. "Impact of thymopentin on the incidence and severity of postoperative infection: a randomized controlled trial." *Br J Surg* 81(2):205–208, 1994.

124 Miller JF. "Immunological function of the thymus." *Lancet* 2:748, 1961.

demonstrated, the importance of the thymus gland was beginning to be revealed.[125]

Once it was discovered that the thymic gland produced these hormone-like effects, several groups of scientists began trying to extract and purify the material from the thymus gland. A number of peptide fragments have been extracted from calf thymus, pig thymus, or from human serum. These peptides are known as thymopoietin, thymulin, and thymic humoral factor, and are thought to be a fragment of a larger molecule localized in the stromal cells of the thymus gland. Despite the modest clinical success of fragmented thymic extracts, the research has indicated that thymic proteins are produced by the epithelial cells of the thymus.

How the Immunity Process Works

Other research has shown that there are two types of lymphocytes: T-lymphocytes and B-lymphocytes. The T-lymphocytes are defined as such because they are derived from or influenced by the thymus. The B-lymphocytes are so called because they are derived from bone marrow. B-lymphocytes are antibody-producing cells that fight bacteria, and the T-lymphocytes provide the primary protection against viral infections and cancer. Malfunction in B-lymphocytes is involved in the immune dysfunction of many autoimmune diseases. Autoimmune diseases are caused by the immune system attacking the body's own tissues. Multiple sclerosis, muscular dystrophy, lupus erythematosis, and possibly juvenile onset diabetes are examples of autoimmune diseases.

By 1971, it had been shown that T-lymphocytes regulated the function and activity of the B-lymphocytes. Recognition of

125 Osaba D, Miller JF. "The lymphoid tissues and immune responses of neonatally thymectomized mice bearing thymus tissue in millipore diffusion chambers." *Jour Exp Med* 119:177, 1964.

the T-lymphocyte's regulatory function in the immune system was important, because it focused on the vital role of the thymic peptides. Research published in 1983 and 1984 brought proof of thymic function for the first time by assembling the varied pieces of the puzzle. Research was based on the theory that the thymus gland is central to proper immune function because it produces protein/ hormones in its epithelium that activate the T-lymphocytes, which in turn promote immunity. The T-lymphocytes also regulate the B-lymphocytes to produce antibodies for fighting infection, and further tell the B-lymphocyte not to attack self tissue.

The lymphocyte in the thymus gland is called a thymocyte and acquires either a CD4 or CD8 characteristic. The CD classification was given to further differentiate the types of T-lymphocytes. Only those thymocytes expressing CD4 or CD8 characteristics are selected to immigrate by way of the thymus gland to the lymphatic system. This differentiation process results in mature lymphocytes that can recognize foreign bodies, viruses, or cancerous cells in the context of major histo-compatible complex hormones. Histo-compatibility refers to the ability of the cells of one tissue to exist in the presence of cells of another tissue, such as would be in the case of a graft or transplant.

The CD4 cells are known as helper cells because they help the immune system by recognizing foreign substances on contact. The CD8 cells are called T-suppressors/cytotoxic or killer cells. They require histo-compatible expression on target cells to be activated to kill them.

Studies have identified at least six types of thymic cells. These particular cells produce interleukin-1 (IL-1), interleukin-4 (IL-4), interleukin-6 (IL-6), thymosin, thymopoietin, and thymulin. These peptides, secreted by the thymus gland, are found to have an effect on T-lymphocyte differentiation and activation. Of these thymic peptides, thymosin, thymulin, thymopoietin, and thymic humoral factor may possibly reach the circulation and act on lymphocytes and tissues at various sites in the human body.

What Do They Each Do?

One of the central questions that remains in studying the thymus gland is to determine the actual role of these peptides. Do they conduct only intrathymic activities, are they secreted by the thymus gland to act on the lymphocytes or tissues in other parts of the human body, or both? If the thymus gland is a hormone-secreting tissue, then alterations in its structure and function may be demonstrated when certain endocrine (hormonal) imbalances exist. Examples might be lack of growth hormone or lack of sex hormone in an individual. Congruously, the function of other tissues may be altered by the presence or absence of thymic peptides. Both types of interactions have been studied, recognized, and proven, suggesting interactive regulatory pathways between the thymus and other endocrine structures.

Dr. Pierpaoli and his coworkers were among the first to identify dependency of the central nervous system's development upon the thymus gland's function. Other studies have established an important interaction between the thymus gland and the development of the pituitary gland in the brain.

The age-related deterioration of the learning and memory abilities also has been linked to atrophy of the thymus gland. However, the mechanism by which the thymus gland affects the central nervous system's cognitive function remains unknown at this time. Test results may reveal a reduction in thymic hormone activity and subsequent deterioration in the human system. In addition to the central nervous system, the thymus gland may also affect functions of other endocrine tissues.

Congenital absence of the thymic gland—beginning from birth—is associated with alterations of the pituitary gland, adrenal gland, thyroid, and ovaries. Drugs that induce hypothyroidism also cause marked atrophy of the thymus gland. T-4 is one type of thyroid hormone. When its levels were reduced following anti-thyroid drug medication treatment, the thymocyte population in the thymus gland was also reduced. Conversely, when T-3, a type of thyroid hormone, was administered in mice, multiple facilitating effects on thymus function were produced. Those effects included increased weight and cell population, as well as enhanced thymocyte production.

Within thirty days following surgery, removal of the pituitary gland resulted in a 50 percent reduction in both thymic gland weight and concentration of the peptide known as thymosin. During the last twenty-five years, at least five separate and distinct thymus peptides/fractions have been isolated and analyzed for T-lymphocyte regulating properties. These are thymosin, thymulin, thymopoietin, thymic humoral factor (THF), and thymic protein-A.

Thymosin

Thymosin (TF) is a group of low molecular-weight peptides extracted from bovine, or cow, thymus. Thymosin has displayed stimulatory effects on T-lymphocyte-mediated immunity. It increased lymphocyte activity and enhanced IL-6 production in spleen cells (IL-6, or interleukin-6, is a protein made by the lymphocyte.). Thymosin had a stimulating effect on luteinizing hormone and gonadotropin-releasing hormone, both pituitary hormones, in studies of pituitary tissues. The release of another pituitary hormone known as prolactin, as well as human growth hormone and adrenal corticotropin (ACTH), are increased by in vitro thymosin studies. Luteinizing hormone was not increased by thymosin in vitro.

Thymulin

Thymulin is a peptide extracted from porcine (pig) thymus tissue. It affects the differentiation of immature bone marrow cells in the function of T-lymphocytes. This thymic peptide stimulates CD8 killer cell lymphocyte activity in the spleen cell cultures obtained from old mice, but not young mice. The serum level of thymulin decreases with age, and coincides with thymus atrophy.

Thymulin requires zinc for full biological activity. Patients who suffer from Crohn's disease, a type of autoimmune intestinal disease, or acute lymphobiastic leukemia, are zinc deficient. They also have a reduction in thymulin activity. All young and old rats had an increase in circulating thymulin levels in response to administration of growth hormone and thyroid peptide injections.

Thymic Humoral Factor (THF)

Thymic humoral factor is an extract of calf thymus. Interleukin-2 (IL-2) is a protein manufactured by lymphocytes. It was enhanced by the influence of THF in spleen cell cultures. Peripheral blood obtained from patients with chronic hepatitis B and viral infections responded to THF with increased production of IL-2. This suggests a possible antiviral role for this thymic peptide, and is one of the reasons we should replace thymic fractions as we move into more mature adulthood after our first two decades.

Thymopoietin (Thymopentin)

Thymopoietin is a peptide extracted from bovine thymus gland. It thoroughly enhances T-lymphocyte differentiation and the effect of function on mature T-lymphocytes. Thymopentin is a protein derivative of thymopoietin, which has the same stimulatory effect on mature cells in the thymus gland.

Thymic Protein-A

Thymic protein-A was discovered in 1983 by Dr. Terry Beardsley. It is a specific protein isolated from a cloned line of epithelial calf thymus cells, which demonstrated immune stimulatory properties similar to those previously obtained by extracts. He called this protein thymic protein-A. It is a five hundred-amino acid chain.

Later, Dr. Esther Hays, in collaboration with Dr. Beardsley, demonstrated that this protein is produced by the human thymus. They transplanted human thymus epithelial cells into the kidneys of mice with no thymus glands. The mice then demonstrated an immune response by living outside a sterile environment without developing infection.[126]

In 1998, the FDA approved HGH for use in humans infected with HIV virus because studies showed results paralleled those seen in animal models, in which restoration of the immune response was demonstrated by resolution of infection, increase in white blood count, and increase in lymphocytes and T-cells.

Thymic peptide replacement can help atrophy of the thymus gland (brought on by the aging process) in the same way diabetics use insulin. The technology now exists to produce these proteins in their natural, intact states. The recent introduction of these proteins in adult humans could have a profound effect on the aging process by restoring the body's natural ability to defend itself from disease and cancers. The thymus gland produces dozens of these proteins, and each one may have a specific purpose in human health and aging. Thymic protein-A is the first of these native, intact, biologically active proteins to become commercially available through sublingual administration. Further research is expected to deliver the other thymic proteins

---

126 Hays E, Beardsley T. "Immunologic effects of human thymic stromal graft and cell lines." *Clin Immunol Immunopath* 33:381, 1984.

without having to inject them parenterally, as they are denatured when ingested.

Thymic protein-A has been shown to stimulate immune response. It activates a specific T-cell, the T-4 (helper) cell, because it has the correct shape to fit the proper receptor site on the T-4 cell and program it to perform its vital immune regulatory functions. The T-4 (helper) cell is responsible for patrolling the body for invading organisms or foreign cells, such as cancer cells. Once activated by thymic protein-A, the T-4 (helper) cell has the ability to identify the invader and signal a response from a specific T-cell, the T-8 (killer) cell, by producing immune proteins called interleukins or interferons. After receiving signals from the T-4 (helper) cell, the T-8 (killer) cell goes to the infection or cancer site and destroys the viral invaders or cancer cells. Thymic protein-A is safe and is available in nutritional supplement form as an immune system stimulant and as part of an antiaging protocol.[127]

Thymic Supplementation

Various studies suggest that the thymus gland and thymic substances contribute to human immunity, the neuroendocrine system, the reproductive system, and the development of the central nervous system. Additionally, alteration in the status of the thyroid, adrenal and pituitary glands, and the kidneys have affected the structure and function of the thymus gland.

Results indicate that the presence of thymic peptides in circulation can have an effect on a variety of other organ systems. Studies include those showing thymic peptides' therapeutic

---

127 Beardsley T, Pierschbacher M, Wetzel GD, Hays EF. "Induction of T-cell maturation by a cloned line of thymic epithelium (TEPI)." *Proc Natl Acad Sci* 80:6005, 1983.

action in atopic dermatitis, rheumatoid arthritis, the prevention of diabetes, and, surprisingly, schizophrenia.[128]

All five preparations we have identified are now commercially available. In all of the studies performed so far, the individual thymic peptides and thymic formulas appear to be safe, causing no unpleasant side effects or adverse reactions. Because several of the thymic peptides are considered by the FDA to be dietary supplements, they are not regulated substances and are available for purchase at most health food stores. Others require a prescription.

Because the research is still in a fairly early stage, your doctor should be notified if you take a thymic supplement so that he or she can monitor your levels and protect your overall health. You should also be aware that, in order to get any benefit from the thymic peptides, you must have enough vitamins, minerals, and enzymes in your body. In fact, the thymic formula is inactive without these other ingredients. For many people, this means taking a multivitamin supplement. A good one should include B complex vitamins, vitamins E and C, selenium, zinc, beta-carotene, and various amino acids.[129]

---

128 Stiller MJ, Shupack JL, Kenny C, et al. "A double-blind, placebo controlled clinical trial to evaluate the safety and efficacy of thymopentin as an adjunctive treatment in atopic dermatitis." *J Am Acad Dermatol* 30(4):597–602, 1994.

Sundal E, Bertelletti D. "Thymopentin treatment of rheumatoid arthritis." *Arzneimittel-Forschung* 44(10):1145–1149, 1994.

Yamanouchi T, Moromizato H, Kojima S, et al. "Prevention of diabetes by thymic hormone in alloxan-treated rats." *Eur J Pharmacol* 257(1–2):39–46, 1994.

Govorin NV, Stupina OP. "Use of thymic peptide thymalin in the complex treatment of therapy-resistant schizophrenia." *Zh Nevropatol Psikhiatr Im S S Korsakova* 90(3): 100–103, 1990.

129 Danese C, Zavattaro E, Calisi L, Marciano F, Perego MA. "Long-term thymopentin treatment in systemic scleroderma." *Curr Med Res Opin* 13(4):195–201, 1994.

THE SYMPHONY

Remember the magic the first time you heard a full symphony orchestra play one of the classics? This work of art is the outcome of balance and order. We may not see the workings of each individual instrument, and we aren't aware of every single note that is played by the orchestra, but we are aware of how beautiful the music sounds, how it moves us, and how we feel; we are aware of the overall performance.

It is the same with our bodies. When everything is in balance, we don't think about how pregnenolone helps our brain function, or the biological mechanisms by which thyroid gives us energy. We simply enjoy the performance of our healthy bodies.

The final effect of total hormone gene therapy is how you feel and function. When you are able to play with your grandchildren for hours at a time and not tire, when you can go back to school and earn a new degree, when you lose fat and find that you can run twice as far, and when you simply feel good about life, you are experiencing the results of a renewed and balanced system.

CHAPTER 13

~

Finding a Physician

THE DOCTOR CAN MAKE THE DIFFERENCE

We have discussed how powerful total hormone gene therapy can be and have shown the wonderful results users experience by bringing their hormone levels up to the optimum. HGH patients, for example, can lose body fat and gain strength while lowering their cholesterol. They strengthen their heart and lungs and greatly improve the functions of the immune system. The kidneys, liver, and digestive system are rejuvenated and may again function like the organs of a younger person. The brain also tends to work better, with improved memory, acuity, and mood. HGH improves the libido and gives greater overall physical energy. It works the wonders of plastic surgery by erasing fine lines and wrinkles, tightening and thickening skin, and even improves the quality and color of hair.

Countless studies, as well as our results from the Palm Springs Life Extension Institute, have proven beyond a doubt the miraculous antiaging and health-giving benefits of HGH and total hormone gene therapy. But as wonderful as HGH is, it is still a potent prescription drug and must be prescribed and administered by a trained physician. Allowing a doctor to evaluate your hormone levels and prescribe an individualized hormone replacement program is essential for a safe and effective return to health.

In order to begin HGH treatment or total hormone gene therapy, you must first find a qualified antiaging and longevity physician who specializes in total hormone gene therapy. This is harder than finding a good orthopedic surgeon, because HGH replacement and total hormone gene therapy are still fairly new treatments. Many doctors have not kept up on the latest advances in this area and may be unwilling to prescribe this hormone.

WHAT TO LOOK FOR

Whenever you begin a new job, you spend several weeks being trained on specific equipment, or new policies and procedures you will need to know. You can't even work the drive-through at McDonald's without first having been prepared for the job. You wouldn't feel comfortable going into brain or heart surgery if the surgeon holding the knife had never actually graduated from medical school or completed a residency. After all, you wouldn't hire an auto body repairperson to rebuild your car's transmission.

In the same manner, you should only trust your physical well-being and lifespan to an individual who has been specifically trained in longevity medicine, especially hormone replacement therapy. As intelligent and skilled as your family doctor may be, he or she is probably not trained in the specifics of hormone replacement and may not be best qualified to aid you in your fight against aging.

There are some basic characteristics to look for and issues to consider when finding a doctor for this treatment. You should find a physician who believes that aging is a disease that can be treated, one who has successfully prescribed hormone replacement in the past, and one who uses the treatment personally, if appropriate. This doctor should be able to effectively determine your needs, monitor your progress, and recommend quality products and supplements.

Finally, seek out a doctor who is on the cutting edge of hormone and antiaging research and can keep you updated on the latest developments in this new and exciting field.

A Doctor Who Believes Aging is a Treatable Disease

Because the study of antiaging and longevity medicine is still a fairly new field, you may experience some difficulty in locating a qualified doctor. There are specific things to look for. First, visit your doctor and tell him or her of the fatigue, weight gain, loss of libido, and decline in mental ability you may have noticed in recent years. If your doctor's response is something to the effect of, "This is perfectly normal for a person of your age," or "What do you expect? You're getting older," you need to walk out of that office and keep looking for adequate medical help.

There are still physicians and other health care providers who view aging as a normal and inevitable part of life. Unfortunately, they also view many of the age-related illnesses we experience as normal. This attitude automatically limits the quality of care you will receive from such a doctor. If your physician cannot see or does not believe that the physical symptoms you are describing are all signs of a disease that needs to be treated, keep searching for help.

On the other hand, if your doctor believes aging is a disease, then you're one step closer. If he or she also believes that this disease, although not yet curable, is treatable, then you may have found a physician you can work with. Before proceeding with treatment, however, make sure any doctor you are considering meets the following additional criteria.

A Doctor Who Has Successfully Used Total Hormone Gene Therapy

If you want to begin any kind of hormone replacement therapy, be sure that your doctor of choice has previously prescribed and administered hormones to a wide range and large number of adult patients. If the only hormone replacement your physician has prescribed is estrogen for post-menopausal women, he or she will probably not have the background and experience to help you bring all your other hormone levels up to their optimal levels.

Finding a doctor with this qualification will probably be more difficult than finding one who believes aging is a disease. Antiaging hormone therapy is still very new, and some hormones—specifically human growth hormone—were not approved for adult use until recently. This fact alone will limit the number of physicians who have a great deal of experience with the hormone. In that case, it may be more important to look at the current number of hormone replacement patients this physician is treating rather than his or her history of treatment. Look for a doctor who is currently treating at least forty patients with antiaging hormone replacement therapy.

A Doctor Using the Therapy

Another telling sign of the ability of your doctor to effectively prescribe a hormone replacement therapy is whether or not the physician uses the treatment personally. Doctors are far from immortal. Like the rest of us, any antiaging or longevity medicine physician you may consult will typically have experienced the negative results of naturally declining hormone levels (unless your doctor is Doogie Howser).

If the doctor has successfully prescribed hormone replacement, then he or she will undoubtedly have seen the benefits of treatment on patients and should also be able to attest to them personally. After all, you want to be treated by doctors who believe in the therapy enough to use it themselves. If a physician doesn't have that much confidence in the therapy, then find one who does.

At the Palm Springs Life Extension Institute, we have not only based our conclusions about HGH and hormone therapy on the data from our patients, we also have experienced the benefits of hormone replacement firsthand. As doctors and administrators of the treatment, we are also patients, and we use and test all the hormones we prescribe. And we are certainly not unique in this aspect.

We feel it is important for the public to realize just how many doctors are using the therapy. These doctors not only recommend hormone therapy for their patients, but they have seen the medical and personal proof to believe that hormone rejuvenation is the key to staying young and healthy.

If your physician is truly committed to longevity medicine, this will be reflected in his or her lifestyle. The doctor of choice should try hard to make a healthy diet and appropriate exercise part of his or her antiaging and longevity regimen and would strongly encourage patients to do the same.

A Doctor with Proven Procedures for Determining Hormone Levels

You should also look for a physician who can effectively determine your hormone levels. This is fairly easy to do, since most hormone levels can be accurately determined with only a simple blood test.

But here again, an established, proven testing procedure is very important. For example, measuring for IGF-1 to determine HGH levels is a bit complicated, and if a lab or physician is not familiar with this type of testing, there can be significant discrepancies in the outcome. A doctor experienced with finely tuned hormone replacement and balancing will also usually use just one laboratory that has proven itself to be accurate. For the careful, individualized treatment that you want, your lab tests should be consistent. Your doctor should also conduct a comprehensive physical exam using tests like those mentioned in our discussion on biologic age.

As was discussed earlier, there is no set standard dosage for hormone replacement. No two human bodies are identical, and each of us has varying physical needs. The recommended hormone treatment depends on the individual, his or her goals and needs, and the specific results of the blood and physical exams. Once your physician has this information, he or she can tailor a hormone replacement treatment specifically designed for your greatest safety and benefit.

A Doctor Who Will Monitor Your Progress

Another important reason for accurate initial testing is that it gives you and your doctor something concrete by which to measure your progress. If, when compared with initial observations, your body fat decreases, your skin quality improves, and you can exercise more, then the treatment is working for you. Comparing the change in blood hormone levels is also essential in monitoring the success and safety of the therapy. This evaluation needs to be done on a regular basis to guarantee that hormones reach their optimal levels, stay constant, and do not get too high.

With hormone replacement therapy, your hormone levels may still change according to physical activity changes and the regeneration and rejuvenation of your organs. The physician must monitor them closely to determine any dose modifications that may be needed for you to reach your optimal levels. A physician still needs to be involved to safely monitor the levels of all the hormones in the body. Many of the hormones work synergistically, and as some levels rise, you may need less of other hormone supplements. Regular monitoring is also important in following the changing hormonal status of certain diseases, such as diabetes.

We've seen the importance of close physician involvement in the cases of patients who come to the Palm Springs Life Extension Institute for treatment. For example, the antiaging hormone DHEA is available for purchase without a prescription. Many people, eager to take advantage of its benefits, have self-prescribed the supplement.

We've seen several patients who, because of the benefits they've experienced with DHEA, come to the Palm Springs Life Extension Institute to be treated with HGH as well. In our standard preliminary testing, we discovered that many of the men who had been self-prescribing DHEA had an enlarged prostate gland. The problem was that many of the over-the-counter supplements were formulated too high, or patients were taking too much. In either case, these individuals were getting more hormone than they needed or could use. As a result, they experienced negative side effects.

We have also seen cases of doctors who, without monitoring their patients' blood hormone levels, repeatedly prescribed estrogen without progesterone for post-menopausal women who have had hysterectomies, only to find that they have increased the risk of their patients developing fibrocystic breast disease or breast cancer.

The competent and experienced physician will regularly test and closely monitor your hormone levels and adjust the dosage to find the treatment that will bring your hormones to their youthful peaks, giving you the greatest possible benefit.

A Doctor Who Can Recommend Quality Hormone Manufacturers and Pharmacies

The antiaging medicine doctor of choice would ideally have a recommended brand of hormone supplement or a specific pharmacy that he or she trusts. Again, with DHEA we have seen that some of the over-the-counter varieties are not properly formulated, often containing less DHEA than the label states. Many of these formulations are also fast-acting, meaning that the hormone does not stay in the system long enough for the body to experience the full benefit. Worse, surges of excess DHEA may result in elevated levels of harmful metabolites in the body. A properly formulated DHEA supplement from a quality pharmacy will be slow-releasing and therefore better able to mimic the body's natural production, bringing your hormones to their optimal levels.

This standard of excellence is necessary with all hormone supplements. The quality of the supplement is vital to the efficacy of the hormone in the body. Technology has advanced to the point where essentially every hormone can be safely manufactured in a laboratory, producing a molecule that is virtually identical to the hormones found in a healthy body. Because they are exact copies, these manufactured hormones are often referred to as natural supplements. Despite this natural option, some physicians still prescribe synthetic designer hormones that are not physiologically or biologically identical to the ones the body produces.

There are companies that produce natural hormones, and pharmacies that distribute quality hormone supplements. These pharmacies are the source of choice for your hormone replacement therapy supplements. A qualified antiaging and longevity medicine physician should be able to point you toward them.

A Doctor Who Will Train You to Supplement

Many hormone supplements have specific instructions for effective use. For example, thyroid hormones are to be taken in the morning, while melatonin should be taken at night, although sometimes in the morning as well, depending on the individual's circadian rhythm. If a patient is not properly trained to use supplemental hormones, he or she simply will not receive the total potential benefit. It is essential to find a doctor who will be able to adequately train you in the best use of all your hormone supplements.

A Doctor Who Keeps Up with Research

Seek out a doctor who is on the cutting edge of antiaging and longevity research and can keep you updated on the latest developments. Revolutionary research is ongoing, and this may well be the decade that sees dramatic changes in longevity for any number of reasons. Ask your doctor what he or she knows about telomeres and antioxidant therapy. It would also be to your advantage to find a doctor who is on the cutting edge of hormone gene therapy research. This is a new medical field, and there is still a great deal to learn.

Research is constantly informing us of the latest advances in hormone therapy, as well as improved methods of administration. In only a few short years, we have learned a great deal about the longevity gene telomerase and its relationship to hormones, and about hormone replacement and the specific antiaging benefits of melatonin, DHEA, and HGH. This rate of discovery is likely to increase in coming years, and in order to receive the greatest benefit from your treatment, you need to be kept well informed of all the latest developments.

A good way to test your physician in this regard is to go in for your first visit with a detailed list of questions. This will require some amount of homework on your part, but if you're reading this book, you've already got a good start. Learn all that you can about hormone replacement therapy and the specific hormones you will probably be using, and then go to your doctor with explicit questions and any concerns that you may have. If the physician can't adequately answer all your questions, or satisfactorily address your concerns, then you may think twice before signing on for his or her treatment.

A Doctor Who Will Continue to be Accessible

Finally, make sure your doctor continues to be accessible. As your treatment continues, you will probably have even more questions, which you should be able to talk over with your doctor or a trained member of his or her staff. Doctor accessibility is not only helpful for responding to your concerns, but also in monitoring your progress, and it is a good indication of your doctor's respect for you as a patient and as a person.

DOES PALM SPRINGS LIFE EXTENSION INSTITUTE MEASURE UP?

At the Palm Springs Life Extension Institute, we try hard to meet or exceed these criteria and provide our patients with the best possible service and treatment. The Institute was founded on the belief that aging is a disease that can be treated, and our efforts are devoted to developing new and better ways to battle the disease.

We have treated more than one thousand growth hormone-replacement patients and prescribe other hormones as well. We have the experience to recommend the best and safest treatments available. Our large research base keeps us on the cutting edge of HGH therapy, and we are constantly searching through new studies and research that help us improve the quality of the services we provide.

We were the first in the United States to use HGH on adults. We were the first to discover and patent the benefits of total hormone gene therapy. We were the first to understand that HGH is not the only hormone that decreases with age and needs to be balanced. We were also the first to recommend replacement of thymic peptides and discover the best site for application of testosterone gel.

We have developed a procedure that is effective and convenient for age-related hormone deficiencies. One centralized lab does bloodwork for patients all across the nation, eliminating the confusion using multiple labs can often result in. Patients can have their blood tested in their hometowns and then sent to the lab for evaluation. A sample prescription for blood tests for men and women is included in Appendix C.

If results indicate hormone deficiencies, the patient makes one trip to our institute. During this visit, the patient receives a complete physical exam and biological age testing that will be used to measure age reversal. Only then can we determine an effective course of treatment.

At this time, we also train the patient on the proper dose and administration of each hormone, sending him or her home with prescriptions and written guidelines. We also recommend the use of one centralized mail order pharmacy to obtain all the hormones prescribed in the therapy. We have tested all products from this pharmacy, have approved them, and we know exactly how well they work.

Once patients are on the program, we monitor their progress, initially every month, until optimal hormone levels are reached.

Then we monitor every six months, all without the patients ever having to leave their hometowns. Again, blood samples can be drawn locally and sent to the lab, and then on to our doctors for evaluation.

We are constantly seeking ways to improve our procedures and the quality of our care to make it increasingly convenient for more and more people to experience the full benefits of hormone replacement.

SELF-MONITORING

No matter which doctor or treatment program you choose, it is important for you to personally monitor your own progress. Even the most involved physician can't be with you all day, every day, and will not be able to know the changes you will feel. Self-monitoring is important in detecting any negative side effects. If you begin to have a less-than-positive reaction to any treatment, let your physician know immediately. Then the therapy can be adjusted to eliminate the problem.

Self-monitoring is also important in keeping track of your improvements. When you begin a treatment program, it would be a good idea to record how you feel physically and what you've noticed about the age-related changes of your body and mind. For example, if you used to be able to run six or seven miles a day, but can now manage ten, write it down. If you've noticed that your skin is smoother and less wrinkled than it was last birthday, or that you are carrying less fat around the middle or on your thighs, you should indicate that as well. Then take this account and add to it as you progress on the treatment.

Many patients keep a journal, recording the physical changes and improvements as they occur, or take photographs of themselves at different points during the treatment (you'll really be able to see the changes if you take photographs of yourself in a swimsuit). Recording these changes can be helpful for your physician and will give you an accurate idea of how you're responding to your therapy. Many patients find it incredible to look back and compare themselves before hormone replacement to how they look and feel after only six months of treatment.

CHAPTER 14

Eating for Youth and Health

LONGEVITY INFLUENCED BY DIET

Even if the new life-extending enzyme telomerase was available to us tomorrow, there would still be differences in the length of the lives that each of us would live. One of the most significant factors that would determine those differences would be our individual choice of diet. From the time we first went to grade school, we've heard from our parents and teachers about the importance of a balanced diet. Science has jumped on the bandwagon, insisting that what we eat is vital to well-being, disease prevention, and longevity. It's about time they caught up.

The reality of food and its different ingredients, good and bad, is that almost everything is essential to maintaining a healthy body. We need types of sugar and carbohydrates for energy. We need protein to build muscle and bone. We even need fat, partly to synthesize cholesterol-based hormones like DHEA, pregnenolone, testosterone, progesterone, and estrogen. And while cholesterol has a bad reputation in healthy eating, it is nonetheless vital to the production of all the steroidal hormones and vitamin D, and for helping the body absorb calcium. It is also a necessary ingredient in the myelin sheath, the fatty coating that protects our nerves, including those of the spinal cord and the brain. In fact, people who have extremely low levels of cholesterol also have an increased risk of cancer and mental illness.

For many of these ingredients, though, a little goes a long way. As in the case of fat or sugar, we don't need much, or we only need a certain kind. But we certainly can't cut them out of our diet entirely.

The difficulty lies in calculating just how much of certain foods we should eat. We have some basic guidelines given to us by the U.S. Department of Agriculture, but in reality, this is a rough estimate. Just as hormone levels differ from person to person, our nutritional needs also depend on who we are, our age, gender, and body composition, so the help of a knowledgeable physician is vital.

A doctor should be able to sit with you and, by learning your age, gender, weight, and metabolism level, personalize a diet for your optimal physical performance. A good diet outline would include information about how much protein, fat, carbohydrates, and sugar you need (or need to avoid), as well as the levels of supplemental vitamins and minerals you should be getting every day. Your nutritional evaluation should also indicate the ideal overall caloric intake for your individual needs.

Physician involvement is important when you consider that hormone therapy (particularly HGH treatment) speeds up the rate of cell growth and tissue repair, therefore using up more nutrients. If you are nutrient poor, the hormones will not be able to do their job as well. A monitored diet also maximizes the benefits of hormone replacement by outlining specific, individual nutritional and caloric needs.

CALORIC RESTRICTION

When some people see the incredible body fat loss and muscle gain they experience through hormone gene therapy, they think, "Finally I can eat what I want and as much as I want." Though it is true that many patients do find that they can eat more than they used to and not gain weight, they still need to keep in mind that one of the most proven therapies in longevity medicine is caloric restriction.

Research has shown that restricting the number of calories we consume is another way to extend life. Since then, the experiments have been reproduced using rats, mice, and rhesus monkeys with similar results.

A 1991 study showed that dietary restriction may work by slowing the aging of the pineal gland. Rats who were on a 40% restricted diet displayed melatonin levels that were twice as high as those in the control group (those who were allowed to eat as much as they would naturally). One year later, another study looked at the effects of dietary restrictions on serum levels of insulin-like growth factor-1. Young mice on the restricted diet initially showed slightly lower-than-normal levels of IGF-1. But by the time these same mice reached old age, their IGF-1 levels were just as high as those of young, healthy control mice.[130]

These studies also indicated that calorie-restricted animals had fewer age-related illnesses, maintained better cardiovascular fitness and immune response, and developed only 25 percent of the tumors of the animals in the control group. They had sleeker coats,

130 Sonntag WE, Lenham JE, Ingram RL. "Effects of aging and dietary restriction on tissue protein synthesis: relationship to plasma insulin-like growth factor-1." *J Gerontol* 47(5):B159–163, 1992.

Stokkan KA, Reiter RJ, Nonaka KO, et al. "Food restriction retards aging of the pineal gland." *Brain Res (Neth)* 545(102):66–72, 1991.

brighter eyes, and normalized levels of blood glucose. The benefits were also visible on a cellular level, since caloric restriction reduced the amount of damage to the individual cells and DNA.[131]

In studies comparing fully fed animals with calorie-restricted animals, the following incidences of disease were observed:

	Fully Fed	Caloric Restricted
Breast cancer	40%	2%
Lung cancer	60%	30%
Liver cancer	64%	0%
Leukemia	65%	10%
Kidney disease	100%	36%
Vascular disease	63%	17%

MAXIMUM LIFESPAN, AVERAGE LIFESPAN

Before we discuss caloric restrictions in humans, we need to understand something about statistics. We hear report after report about how short the average lifespan was hundreds of years ago and how much improved that is today. For example, we might say, "In ancient Rome, the average lifespan was twenty-two years, but today, at least in Western countries, it's about seventy-five years." The term *average lifespan* actually refers to the age at which half the population is dead and half the population is still alive.

131 Kemnitz JW, Roecker EB, Weindruch R, et al. "Dietary restriction increases insulin sensitivity and lowers blood glucose in rhesus monkeys." *Am J Physiol* 266(4):E540–547, 1994.

Turturro A, Blank K, Murasko D, Hart R. "Mechanisms of caloric restriction affecting aging and disease." *Ann NY Acad Sci* 719:159–170, 1994.

Weindruch R, Walford RL, Fligiel S, Guthrie D. "The retardation of aging in mice by dietary restriction: longevity, cancer, immunity and lifetime energy intake." *J Nutr* 116(4):641–654, 1986.

This contrasts with *maximum lifespan*, which is the documented upper limit of years of life for the most elderly of the human species. For human beings, the maximum lifespan is about one hundred twenty to one hundred thirty years. This hasn't changed much since Roman times. In ancient Rome, a lot of people did die at much younger ages because of illnesses we now can cure, or from diseases we now know how to prevent. But there were always a few people who lived to ages as high as one hundred thirty years.

When we talk about caloric restriction extending the life of mice, we mean that the maximum lifespan for mice on a normal diet is about forty-one months. This is the oldest age mice ever reach and equates to being a one hundred twenty-year-old human. But on a calorie-restricted diet, the maximum lifespan for mice was extended to fifty-six months. That's the equivalent of pushing the upper limit to more than one hundred fifty human years!

DOES IT WORK IN HUMANS?

Does caloric restriction have a similar effect on humans? Well, because this is a longevity study, researchers have not yet been able to determine the effects of caloric restriction over a sixty- to seventy-year period. But a study published in 1992 showed the benefits of caloric restriction on the scientists who participated in the Biosphere 2 project.[132] The scientists lived for two years inside a self-contained laboratory and home where they had to grow and raise their own food. The food they grew was nutrient-rich, but their caloric intake was 30 percent to 35 percent less than that of the average American.

---

132 Walford RL, Harris SB, Gunion MW. "The calorically restricted low-fat nutrient-dense diet in Biosphere 2 significantly lowers blood glucose, total leukocyte count, cholesterol, and blood pressure in humans." *Proc Natl Acad Sci USA* 89(23):11533–37, 1992.

After the study, team members had lower blood pressure, cholesterol, and fasting blood sugar levels than they had before entering Biosphere 2. One year later, after a normal diet, the levels were still low. This evidence convinced many researchers that the benefits of caloric restriction seen in rodents would also apply to humans.

By *caloric restriction*, we don't mean dieting, and we don't mean starving yourself. If starving yourself worked, then semi-starved populations in developing countries would have longer maximum lifespans than we do, which they do not. They are caloric restricted, but they are also malnourished. Effective caloric restriction is to have the absolute highest quality nutrition in the fewest number of calories possible. Ideally, your caloric limit—determined with the help of a doctor who considers all of your individual characteristics—would give your body everything it needs, and only that.

MORE CALORIES, MORE FREE RADICALS

If the decline in hormones such as HGH and the shutdown of the longevity gene telomerase is the number one cause of aging, guess what's number two? The answer is free radical damage and destruction, or oxidative stress as it's sometimes called. The more food we take in, the more energy we need to digest it and convert it into calories. The more energy we need, the more oxygen we have to burn, since we use oxygen as fuel. The splitting of the O_2 molecule for energy is like setting off an oxygen bomb. The more bombs we set off, the more damage we do to our cells through oxidative stress. Debris from the bomb's explosion are called free radicals.

Oxidative stress caused by free radicals is an unavoidable part of being human. It is the price we pay for breathing. We create free radicals inside our bodies as a byproduct of the oxygen-burning processes that create energy essential to the functioning of each individual cell. We are also surrounded by these damaging molecules wherever we go and whatever we do. Free radicals are present in pollution, smog, radiation from sunlight, and cigarette smoke. Other lifestyle factors, such as lack of exercise, a poor diet, and too much stress increase the oxidative damage we do to our bodies.

Every time we overload our bodies with poor quality food or more food than we need and can use, we open ourselves up to the damaging effects of free radicals. Free radicals are toxic and dangerous scavengers because their physical makeup includes one or more unpaired electrons. This makes them highly reactive because, in order to pair off their lone electrons, they scavenge electrons from other molecules They attack the DNA in our cells and destroy cell membranes, causing a chain reaction of constant cell damage. They break off cell membrane proteins, destroying the cell's identity; they harden cell membranes, leading to brittle and nonfunctional cells; they expose sensitive genetic material, leaving the DNA open to mutation or destruction; and they burden the immune system by damaging immune cells. In turn, the damage causes, hastens, or encourages growth of a host of chronic diseases, collectively known as oxidative stress.

Free radical damage plays a part in the development of serious diseases, including arthritis, cataracts, heart disease, diabetes, cancer, and aging. The unchecked spread of free radicals can also cause wrinkles, age spots, and stiff joints. This spread of oxygen-induced cellular damage in our body is similar to the spread of rust on metal. Rust spreads until it destroys the structure and strength of the metal. Similarly, the spread of free radicals weakens the body. As the system becomes more and more damaged, the free radicals spread even more quickly because our bodies are weakened and therefore less effective at neutralizing them. Oxidative stress contributes significantly to the negative effects of aging.

ANTIOXIDANTS ARE THE ANTIDOTE

To stop free radicals from aging us on a cellular level, our body uses antioxidants, micro-nutrients that easily react with oxygen to neutralize the free radicals, ending their trail of destruction and removing them from the body entirely. Some of the most common antioxidants are vitamins C, E, beta-carotene, selenium, and melatonin.

In an ideal world, we would all live healthy lives, without dangerous toxins such as alcohol and tobacco, and without the dangers of too much sunlight and stress. We would obtain the important antioxidants in sufficient amounts as part of a normal healthy diet, and oxidative stress would not be a problem.

Unfortunately, we do not live in an ideal world. Instead, we live in one that is more and more polluted and filled with almost constant stress. This stress often comes with skipped meals, meals on the run, and fast-food consumption.

In this imperfect world, many of us have imperfect diets. Recent studies reveal that middle-class people who are leading comfortable lives are taking less than one-fourth of the required amount of vitamins. Another study from 1990 estimated that only 9 percent of Americans eat the recommended five servings a day of fruits and vegetables. This lack of vitamins is a serious health problem today. Even those who eat a healthy diet may not get sufficient amounts of the necessary nutrients because their bodies are not absorbing them properly. Poor absorption can be caused by allergies, laxative and antacid use, protein deficiency, stress, lack of exercise, and simply getting older.

GETTING THE NUTRIENTS WE NEED

It is unlikely, even with good absorption, that we're getting the nutrients we need. Our diet today—even a healthy and balanced one—consists of food that has been grown in pesticide-contaminated soil. It is then packaged, refined, processed, manufactured, cooked, frozen, canned, and often pressed and chopped into a completely unrecognizable form. Each of these steps removes some of the food's natural supply of vitamins and minerals. For example, vitamin E is almost always lost in even the simplest of processes. The absence of vitamin E results in a subsequent loss of vitamin A and beta-carotene of up to 90 percent. Almost all of the essential nutrients are destroyed or lost to some degree during food processing.

A growing number of experts believe that even the most well-balanced, healthy diet on the planet will not provide enough antioxidants to protect us from oxidative damage. The food we eat simply does not provide us with enough of the antioxidant vitamins and minerals to fight off all the bad effects of the free radicals. Studies done in both home and hospital settings show that most of us, particularly as we grow older, simply cannot get enough antioxidants in our diet.[133]

So even with all the wonders of modern medicine we have at our fingertips, we're still losing the war against age with every bite we take. Nutrient-deficient foods, combined with pollution and stress, form an invading army our bodies and modern-day technologies are not yet equipped to do battle with.

ANTIOXIDANT THERAPY

So what can we do to fight the oxidation that threatens to destroy our bodies cell by cell? We are certainly not about to give in to the destructive forces of the free radicals without a fight. Since diet

133 Schmuck A, Ravel A, Coudray C, et al. "Antioxidant vitamins in hospitalized elderly patients: analysed dietary intakes and biochemical status." *Eur J Clin Nutr* 50(7):473–478, 1996.

alone is not sufficient to stop the oxidative damage, more and more doctors are recommending people take dietary supplements.

It can be rather dizzying to walk into a health food store or browse the vitamin aisle of the grocery store and see the conglomeration of supplement pills, capsules, teas, extracts, elixirs, and creams, some bearing strange names. If you were to buy every product in the store that could benefit you, you would spend all your waking hours taking pills and supplements, consuming more than one thousand dollars a day in products. So out of the maze of health-craze products, which do you choose? Which will really be worth your time and money?

It would literally take you hours to sort through the maze of labels to answer these questions. So to give you a starting place in your search for supplements, we have a few recommendations. One thing to keep in mind as you begin taking dietary supplements is that these substances will not work as quickly as medications and drugs you may be using. Dietary supplements are mainly preventive, and as a result, you may not notice an immediate, dramatic change. The improvement will only come with time and perseverance, so be patient.

MULTIVITAMIN AND MINERAL SUPPLEMENTS

The fundamental ingredient in any dietary supplement regimen is a comprehensive multivitamin and mineral combination. The U.S. government has created dietary requirements for most vitamins and minerals. However, these levels were determined by the amount necessary to prevent clinical deficiency syndromes. For optimal health and nutrition, we really need amounts far above the USDA recommended daily allowances. This means taking a fairly high-powered multivitamin and mineral complex.

Vitamins are essential to both the structure and functioning of the body. They operate as coenzymes, which are necessary elements for chemical reactions and energy production. Vitamins are essential to sustaining human life and cannot be manufactured by the body, so we must get them from the food we eat or from a dietary supplement.

There are twenty different kinds of minerals we need for growth and maintenance, and most of these can be found in food. The oceans and soil contain minerals which are absorbed by food that we eat. For example, spinach contains iron, persimmons contain magnesium, and some fruits, especially bananas, contain potassium. However, as we have already discussed, it is difficult to get a well-balanced diet with sufficient levels of nutrients, and it is important to find a supplement that contains an adequate amount of minerals.

Minerals work in combination with enzymes, hormones, vitamins, and transport substances to aid in nerve transmission, muscle conduction, cell permeability, tissue rigidity and structure, blood formation, aid-base balance, fluid regulation, protein metabolism, and energy production. Calcium and phosphorus are essential for maintaining teeth and bone health. Iron is needed to make hemoglobin, which in turn makes blood corpuscles. We also need sulfur for our hair and nails.

Minerals are crucial in maintaining good health, not only physically, but also mentally. For example, potassium is found in our body fluids in a very small amount, but if that amount drops, we may experience irritability, anxiety, and insomnia. Potassium works to soothe agitation of our nerves, and negative side effects can result from low levels. Magnesium deficiency may cause mumbling and overall mental imbalance.

Minerals also provide the body with nutrients used for making hormones. For example, iodine is an essential ingredient in the production of thyroid hormone. In Japan, people take in plenty of iodine by consuming large amounts of kelp, which is a good source of iodine. Those who live a continent away from the sea have traditionally been susceptible to thyroid problems.

Ideally, you will find one multivitamin and mineral supplement that contains the necessary elements. Some of the absolute essentials include vitamin A, beta-carotene, vitamin C, vitamin E, vitamin K, vitamins B1 (thiamin), B2 (riboflavin), B3 (niacin), B6 (pyridoxine), B12, and folic acid. Biotin and pantothenic acid (B5) should also be included. Additionally, the supplement of choice should contain the minerals calcium, chromium, copper, magnesium, manganese, selenium, and zinc. Iron is another fundamental mineral especially essential to women. However, iron supplementation in men can lead to a disease process called hemochromatosis, a disorder that interferes with the body's ability to break down iron, and results in too much iron being absorbed from the gastrointestinal tract, as well as arteriosclerosis, so dietary supplementation of iron is not recommended for men.

Why are these ingredients necessary? There is so much material available it could fill another book, but here we will touch on the benefits of a few of the vitamins and minerals.

ANTIOXIDANTS

We've already explained why antioxidants are important. The antioxidant quality of certain vitamins and minerals is one of the greatest benefits of any multivitamin regimen. The most important antioxidants include beta-carotene, vitamins C and E, and selenium, and, as we will explain below, they do much more than just fight off free radicals. Some of these antioxidants, in particular vitamins C and E, should be taken in extra amounts, in addition to your multivitamin.

Vitamin A

This vitamin promotes good vision, protects the heart and cardiovascular system, boosts the immune system, speeds recovery from respiratory infections, promotes wound healing, slows down the aging process, and prevents and possibly reverses the course of certain forms of cancer. Vitamin A also plays an important role in maintaining healthy skin.

However, excessive intake of vitamin A can lead to hair loss, nausea, scaly skin, bone pain, fatigue, blurred vision, and liver enlargement. For this reason, many prefer to take beta-carotene (provitamin A), which is converted into vitamin A in the liver whenever your body needs it. This makes it an extremely safe source of the needed vitamin A, with none of the adverse side effects.

Beta-Carotene

In addition to doing the work of vitamin A, beta-carotene is a powerful antioxidant. In fact, it can do several things other antioxidants cannot. Beta-carotene can work in areas of low oxygen (such as the capillaries), and is unaffected by its encounters with cancer-causing substances, and can therefore neutralize a larger number of free radicals. In numerous studies, beta-carotene-rich diets have been linked to a decreased risk of cancer and heart disease. Major sources of this nutrient include carrots, squash, broccoli, spinach, apricots, papayas, and other yellow and dark green vegetables. But many researchers believe most people don't get enough beta-carotene, even when they think they are eating large amounts of these foods. Beta-carotene supplements are a good idea and absolutely non-toxic, even when taken at high doses.

Vitamin C

Vitamin C supplements should be taken daily, since this vitamin is instrumental in the well being of more than 300 bodily functions. It is water-soluble, which means the body doesn't store it if it doesn't need it. Vitamin C is stored mainly in the adrenal gland, and if the adrenal gland tires out, it will deplete vitamin C promptly. A severe vitamin C deficiency shows up as scurvy, a disease that claimed the lives of many sailors back in the days of long sea voyages and no fresh rations. Scurvy symptoms include bleeding gums, loosened teeth, dry, rough skin, anemia, joint pain, bruising, and frequent infections. Sufficient vitamin C prevents these symptoms.

Vitamin C is a powerful antioxidant that protects against the harmful effects of cigarette smoke, pollution, toxins, and other free radical-causing agents. It also strengthens the adrenal gland and immune system, helping the body resist infection and stress. One of the other important functions of vitamin C is to improve the absorption of iron, which helps maintain healthy red blood cells. In fact, if you are taking an iron supplement, you should also take vitamin C to make sure your body is able to use all of the iron.

But the primary job of vitamin C is to maintain collagen, a protein necessary for the formation of skin, connective tissue, bones, and teeth. It strengthens the walls of blood vessels and helps our bodies heal faster. A good plan is to take one gram of vitamin C at least three times a day, as we should have at least three grams daily. A few foods that contain vitamin C include broccoli, parsley, oranges, tangerines, lemons, sweet potatoes, kiwis, and strawberries.

Vitamin E

Vitamin E is especially necessary for people who are trying to reduce the amount of fat in their diets. Some studies show that vitamin E intake drastically falls when following a low-fat diet, leaving an individual vulnerable to the damaging effects of free radicals. Vitamin E, a powerful antioxidant, protects the cells from the effects of various toxins, including certain chemotherapy drugs. Vitamin E also protects from free radical skin damage, much of which is caused by exposure to the sun. No doubt you have seen vitamin E included in the ingredient list for many lotions and skin care products. In these combinations, vitamin E can help diminish liver spots, treat acne and burns, prevent scarring, and help reduce the appearance of wrinkles.

Vitamin E is vital to our health for more than cosmetic reasons. It supplies oxygen to the organs and muscles of the body (including the heart), and helps keep our red blood cells healthy. A new study shows that vitamin E supplementation may also prevent or delay the worsening of chronic heart disease in elderly patients by lowering blood insulin levels. Too much sugar in the blood is one of the main risk factors for chronic heart disease.[134]

Selenium

Selenium is another powerful antioxidant that also appears to have cancer-fighting properties. We get selenium from our diet, but content varies according to the concentration of the mineral in the soil where the food was grown. High rates of cancer have been linked to low levels of selenium in the soil, and in areas where soil selenium levels are high, the incidence of cancer is lower. The December 25, 1996, issue of the *Journal of the American Medical Association* told of a study that looked at the effect of selenium supplementation on various types of cancer. The results showed that the selenium group

134 Paolisso G, Gambardella A, et al. "Chronic intake of pharmacological doses of vitamin E might be useful in the therapy of elderly patients with coronary heart disease." *Am J Clin Nutr* 81:848–852, 1995.

had 63 percent less prostate cancer, 58 percent less colon cancer, and 46 percent fewer cases of lung cancer than the placebo group. Overall, the selenium group had a 37 percent reduction in cancer cases, and 50 percent fewer cancer-related deaths.

Selenium also has other powerful characteristics. For example, it has proven successful in treating psoriasis and allergies. Selenium also enhances the activity of specific enzymes, some of which can help repair muscle tissue, including heart muscle tissue, which reduces the risk of a heart attack. Combining selenium with vitamin E appears to be effective in strengthening the immune system. A 1996 study also reported selenium's link to the hormone thyroid. As we discussed earlier, thyroid is a key hormone in fat metabolism in adults. Therefore, by helping activate the thyroid hormone, selenium may play an important role in reducing the amount of fat our bodies store.

Vitamin D

Vitamin D strengthens bones by assisting in the absorption of calcium, particularly as we age. Our bones are created and broken down through the processes of osteoclast and osteoblast. After osteoclasts destroy old bone, cells called osteoblasts allow calcium to settle to create new bone. However, without vitamin D, the precious calcium is expelled from the body.

Vitamin D teams up with adrenal hormones and urges intestines to absorb calcium. Without vitamin D, calcium cannot be used as a building material in our bones. If the bones continue to deteriorate, they become brittle and break easily. Some of our patients have exclaimed, "I only slipped and fell down, and now I have a broken bone!" As the bones continue to deteriorate, you may experience pain in your bones and joints and suffer from lower back pain.

You do not necessarily have to resort to drinking milk for vitamin D. The best kept secret about getting enough vitamin D is to spend a little time in the sun. Vitamin D is produced as sunlight hits your body, and you can get enough of the vitamin for one day if you stay in direct sunlight for just ten minutes, without sunscreen. Vitamin D can also be found in liver, sardines, tuna, bonito, egg yolks, and mushrooms.

Vitamin B6

Hormones and vitamin B6 form an inseparable partnership in our bodies. Vitamin B6 is used in the necessary process of converting tryptophan, an essential ingredient in some hormones, into serotonin. Vitamin B6 also allows us to live a regular and rhythmical life by prompting the production of melatonin. Those who smoke, drink alcoholic beverages, and consume large amounts of processed food are especially at risk for low vitamin B6 levels.

Vitamin B6 is found abundantly in bananas, carrots, liver, shrimp, soybeans, avocados, wheat germ, hazelnuts, lentils, salmon, tuna, sunflower seeds, yeast, rice, and dairy products.

Calcium

Of all the minerals, we most often lose calcium. The rule is that the concentration of calcium inside a cell must be one-ten thousandth of the concentration outside the cell. However, many of us are deficient in calcium, especially as we grow older, and this can have an effect not only on our bones but on our hormones. For example, calcium is essential for the secretion of melatonin. Research indicates that nighttime melatonin secretion will increase if you take calcium before going to sleep.

The body's cells absorb only the minimum amount of calcium necessary for proper functioning. If we have low levels of calcium, it will begin to leave our bones and settle inside the brain and blood vessels. Because of this peculiar characteristic of calcium, our body as a whole may lack calcium, while certain organs contain an excess amount of calcium.

Adrenal hormones play an important role in regulating the amount of calcium in the body. If we have low levels of calcium, adrenal hormones will draw the mineral from our bones as needed, and prevent calcium loss from the kidneys. The hormones will also urge the secretion of vitamin D, which helps absorb calcium from the intestinal tract. The adrenal gland will do its best to keep calcium in the body and to raise the concentration of calcium in the blood.

The absorption rate of calcium can actually decrease if we consume too much calcium, so follow your doctor's advice about the right amount for you.

Salt

Salt, which contains sodium, is also an immediate source of minerals. Our body must have sodium for survival; however, we must be cautious because sodium can become an enemy to our hormones. As the body tries to expel excess sodium, body fluid decreases. A hormone called vasopressin is secreted in the pituitary gland of the brain to regulate the body's water content. The brain also secretes a hormone called angiotensin, which causes us to feel thirst so we will drink water to replenish our body's fluids. Even a subtle excess of sodium will affect the complex process of this mechanism. Not only is too much salt damaging to our hormones, it may also trigger high blood pressure. Fewer than five grams of sodium per day would be ideal, but we should limit our intake to no more than ten grams per day. Keep in mind, one teaspoon of salt contains six grams of sodium, or 2,400 milligrams. The recommended daily intake of sodium is 2,500 milligrams for healthy adults. Most of our sodium intake comes from packaged foods, such as potato chips, soups, pre-packaged meals, etc. Always read labels carefully to avoid too much sodium intake!

ADDITIONAL SUPPLEMENTS

We've highlighted only a small number of the vitamins and minerals we recommend, and we've discussed only a few of the benefits of certain vitamins and minerals. Depending on your individual health needs and goals, you may want to take some additional dietary supplements. Vitamins and minerals are a great place to start in boosting your nutritional intake, but there are other supplements that may prove to be lifesavers for some people. This is when the health food store turns into a frightening labyrinth of labels, price tags, and strange-sounding names. Here are a few of the choices we recommend the most.

Grape Seed Extract

Grape seed extract contains a high concentration of a bioflavonoid complex called procyanidolic oligomers (PCO), which acts as a powerful antioxidant—some say fifty times more powerful than vitamin E—that can even cross the blood-brain barrier. It also strengthens collagen and elastin, our body's connective tissue. Bioflavonoids are not manufactured by the body. Because of this, we must get them from the foods we eat or from supplements.

Although bioflavonoids are found in the skins of many fruits, researchers have discovered that the bioflavonoids that come from grape seeds are the most concentrated and have the greatest antioxidant effect. Grape seed extract has proven effective in treating arthritis, allergies, hardening of the arteries, ulcers, gum disease, wrinkles, and spots on the skin, and as part of the prevention of cancer, strokes, and diabetes.

The bioflavonoids in grape seed extract are effective in treating arthritis because of their anti-inflammatory abilities. PCO in particular inhibits the release and synthesis of compounds that promote inflammation. Grape seed extract is effective in treating allergies and colds as it blocks the enzyme that is responsible for the production of histamine. Excess histamine is also what causes stress-induced ulcers in the stomach. By reducing histamine secretion and strengthening the stomach's connective tissue, PCO helps ulcers heal.

In February 1995, the American Heart Association released the results of a study that showed that regular consumption of wine could help keep the heart healthy. Many researchers now believe that these benefits come from the bioflavonoids found in the grapes rather than from the alcohol found in wine. PCO protects against cardiovascular disease by preventing the oxidation of LDL cholesterol (one of the major causes of hardened arteries), and by improving blood vessel elasticity. It also helps keep red blood cells pliable, reducing the risk of blood clots and stroke.

Because it strengthens tissue, grape seed extract helps preserve gum health and protect against tooth decay. Its antioxidant properties also seem to protect the eye from cataracts. Age-related macular degeneration, caused by damage to the retina, is also improved by the antioxidant and collagen-building characteristics of PCO.

Grape seed extract is non-toxic, but its bitterness can sometimes cause nausea or stomach upset. It is water soluble and absorbed into the body within only sixty minutes of consumption.[135]

Ginkgo Biloba

Ginkgo biloba is an herbal extract that comes from the leaves of an ornamental tree often used to decorate parks, city streets, and

135 Hansen C. *Grape Seed Extract: Procyanidolic Oligomers (PCO).* New York: Healing Wisdom Publications, 1995.

yards. Various studies show that Ginkgo biloba can be a powerful therapy for conditions including Alzheimer's disease, asthma, headaches, impotence, and circulatory disorders. It also acts as an antioxidant since it contains bioflavonoids.

Research out of Germany shows that geriatric patients who received Ginkgo biloba extract were more alert and performed better on psychometric tests. They also seemed to be more positive about life. Results of a London study showed that Ginkgo biloba administration also had a positive effect on adult patients with mild to moderate memory loss. These results suggest that Ginkgo biloba extract may be able to delay mental deterioration and reverse some of the disabilities associated with Alzheimer's disease.

Coenzyme Q-10

In this book we have devoted a great deal of time to hormones, and how necessary they are for the proper functioning of the body. But just as we need more than one hormone to keep the entire body healthy, we need other, non-hormone substances to help the body function well. Enzymes are proteins combined with a mineral or vitamin which provide catalysts for every chemical change that takes place in the body. The vitamin portion of the enzyme is usually called the coenzyme.

Coenzyme Q-10 (CoQ10) is found in every cell in the body and helps convert the food we eat into adenosine triphosphate (ATP), the fuel for all our cellular functions. This important role makes CoQ10 essential for the health of the entire body. One researcher found that levels of CoQ10 decline by as much as 80% as we age. Animal studies indicate that low levels of CoQ10 are linked to the age-related decline in immune system functioning.

Low levels of CoQ10 have also been associated with heart disease and liver trouble. That is because these two organs have the highest natural concentrations of CoQ10. They both need great amounts of the coenzyme to perform their highly energy-dependent functions. Research suggests that 50 percent to 75 percent of cardiac patients are deficient in CoQ10, which helps maintain the constant pumping action of the heart. Without it, the tissue and the muscle action weaken. Studies show that treatment with CoQ10 increases treadmill exercise tolerance in cardiac patients. Also, after four weeks of treatment, 53 percent of congestive heart failure patients were asymptomatic. CoQ10 also helps maintain healthy blood pressure by correcting the metabolic abnormalities that cause hypertension.

By energizing the liver and helping it operate at maximum efficiency, CoQ10 aids in cleaning dangerous toxins out of the body. This is especially important for individuals who may be taking prescription drugs that can have toxic side effects. The liver is also responsible for the production of a substance called bile that helps to break down the fat stores in the body. This means that CoQ10 can help maintain a healthy body weight. It also restores normal metabolic activities that balance the fat use/storage ratio. In fact, research shows that more than 50 percent of obese individuals are also deficient in CoQ10 and, when on a supplement treatment combined with a restricted diet, study subjects averaged a weight loss of more than twenty-five pounds after only nine weeks.

This particular substance has been used in Japan for decades, and in the United States for the past several years. CoQ10 is generally well tolerated and, aside from a few instances of nausea and diarrhea, shows no serious side effects.[136]

---

136 Lee WH. *Coenzyme Q-10: Is it Our New Fountain of Youth?* New Canaan, Conn.: Keats Publishing, 1987.

PROTEIN

When we eat food that contains protein, the protein is broken down by the digestive organs and converted into a minuscule amount of amino acid. This amino acid is then converted into enzymes, new proteins, or hormones. In order to maintain our hormones, it is therefore imperative for us to consume sufficient amounts of good quality protein. There are eight essential amino acids that we need, and we call these the "essential eight." The protein in wheat, for example, does not contain all eight essential amino acids. The only grain that contains all eight essential amino acids is called quinoa (pronounced keen-wah), which has a light, fluffy texture when cooked and a mild, slightly nutty flavor. It's available in almost every supermarket or specialty store and is easy to prepare.

What is a good example of a balanced diet that contains the essential eight? Let's take a look at a common Japanese breakfast served at inns. The breakfast would consist of white steamed rice, miso soup, and eggs. The white rice lacks only one amino acid called lysine, but the miso soup conveniently provides it. Fresh eggs contain methionine, which is lacking in other breakfast foods. As a whole, the traditional Japanese breakfast provides all eight essential amino acids and is ideal for the formation of good hormones.

With the help of hormones, amino acids are converted into useful protein to be stored as muscle. We call this process *protein anabolism* or *assimilation*. Conversely, the protein stored in muscles can be converted into amino acids. This process is called *protein catabolism*. Various hormones participate in these two processes. In the case of protein anabolism, growth hormone, thyroid hormone, adrenocortical hormone, and male hormones all work together. In the case of protein catabolism, cortisol and adrenaline secreted by the adrenal medulla work together to break down muscle.

Because declining muscle mass is directly linked to an increase in age-related disability, building muscle is another key to staying active and healthy for years. After we stop growing, the process of anabolism, or muscle development, begins to slow down. As we age, the process of catabolism becomes more frequent than that of anabolism. Naturally, our muscles begin to weaken and we become what people call "flabby." Another reason for the slowing down of the process of anabolism is the decrease in secretion of DHEA by the adrenal gland.

The body continues to secrete most of the hormones without a conspicuous drop from the teens all the way to the sixties, but DHEA begins to decrease in our twenties. On the contrary, cortisol, which plays a strong role in catabolism and is secreted by the adrenal gland, does not decrease. This widening gap causes our muscles to age. When a young person eats protein, most of the protein is converted into muscle and blood, but an older person is not so fortunate. The aging of muscles normally begins in a man's forties and fifties, and the average American male loses anywhere from 4.5 to 7.5 kg of muscle between the ages of forty and seventy. The loss of muscle, stamina, and strength is rapid, and is one symptom of andropause. However, andropause is not an inevitable event. We can consume more protein and replace our hormones.

If you are actively training and trying to build muscle mass, you will likely need more protein than what you can get from your diet. If you want that extra protein boost, here are a few suggestions.

Whey Protein

Whey protein is the supplement of choice, because it contains the highest amount of branched-chain amino acids, which provide the building materials for the amino acids alanine, glutamine, and leucine, important to muscle protein synthesis and in preventing the breakdown of muscle protein during exercise.

Leucine

Leucine is the most important branched-chain amino acid, since muscles tend to burn more leucine than any other amino acid. Leucine also promotes the natural release of HGH, thyroid hormone, and insulin. By supplying branched-chain amino acids, you reduce the muscle's need to burn its own proteins during exercise.

Soy Powder

Soy powder is another option, although it does not contain as high a concentration of protein as do supplements like whey. But soy does provide some significant isoflavones, which help prevent cancer and can reduce cholesterol by up to 35 percent. One of the most powerful isoflavones, genistein, has been found to be a potent anti-cancer agent. Genistein acts as an antioxidant, and it also prevents cancer cell multiplication by starving the cells of the nutrients they need to survive. It is well known that residents of the Far East have a low incidence of colon, breast, and prostate cancers, and professionals believe this is due to the large amount of soy in their diets.

Other Protein Supplements

Three other supplements have been shown to help build muscle. Glutamine is the most abundant free amino acid in the muscle, increasing protein synthesis, and preventing the breakdown of protein during exercise. Hydroxymethylbuterate (HMB), a metabolite of the amino acid leucine, also builds muscle and protects it from the damages of weight training. Creatine aids in the production of ATP, which is the body's main energy source, and aids in high-intensity exercises such as weight training and aerobic exercise.[137]

WATER

Most of us would never consider only washing our hands half of the time, or bathing only when it was convenient. In fact, most Americans devote a great deal of time keeping their bodies clean. Ironically, while time and money are dedicated to skin and hair cleanliness, little attention is paid to how clean the *insides* of our bodies are. We know that if we don't bathe or wash our hands, we can get sick. Likewise, without washing our insides, we greatly increase our chances of catching viruses and bacteria.

Keeping our insides clean means keeping our bodies sufficiently hydrated. This is a simple process. It doesn't require expensive supplements or creams. You simply have to drink water. If it makes you feel better, you can even spend a little more and drink only bottled water. But the simple, inexpensive, natural substance we know as water is essential to our physical health, and, sadly, is too often overlooked.

About 70 percent of the human body is water and is essential for everything the body does. All the biochemical reactions in the body take place in water, and nutrients are transported to all parts of the body through liquid. Toxins and wastes are cleaned out by water. Some experts estimate that the average person loses at least two quarts of water each day through the regular biological

---

137 Lamartiniere CA, Moore J, Barnes S, Holland M. " Neonatal genistein chemo prevents mammary cancer." *Proc Soc Exp Biol Med* 208(1):120–123, 1995.

Adlercreutz CH, Goldin BR, Gorbach SL, Hockerstedt KA, Watanabe S, Hamalainen EK, Markkanen MH, Makela TH, Wahala KT. "Soybean phytoestrogen intake and cancer risk." *J Nutr* 125(7):1960, 1995.

processes of perspiration, elimination, and evaporation from the lungs. If we are not replacing this water, the body's functions are hampered. It is recommended that you drink eight to ten eight-ounce glasses of water every day. This requirement increases if you are exercising a lot or live in a hot and dry climate.

Simple, inexpensive water is the key to many aspects of our overall health. Besides transporting nutrients and ridding the body of wastes and toxins, water helps maintain a healthy body temperature. Drinking cold water is an effective way of bringing down a fever. Water also acts as a natural appetite suppressant and weight loss aid, since it helps the body metabolize stored fat. Forget the diet pills. Drink more water.

In addition, you may not need to spend money on laxatives if you drink enough water, since it is a natural cure for constipation. If you drink enough water, you will also have fewer digestive problems and will absorb even more of the nutrients from the foods you eat. Water also is key in maintaining healthy muscle and skin tone.

Some people worry that drinking too much water will cause water retention. In fact, drinking water stimulates the kidneys, reducing water retention. We've all heard that when we are sick we need to drink lots of fluids. But be aware that coffee, soda pop, and alcohol will not give you the same benefits that water will. Drinking water when you have a cold or flu will help flush the virus out of your body, as well as assist the rest of your systems in functioning as best as they can during the illness. Drinking sufficient water can also help prevent illness in the first place.

It can be difficult to keep track of how much water you are drinking during the day, but here is some simple advice to help you meet your body's water needs of at least eight eight-ounce glasses of water a day: never pass a drinking fountain without stopping and taking a drink; have water at your desk at work; carry water in your car with you; and make sure you drink sufficient amounts of water while exercising. Basically, you should carry water around (and drink it, of course) all day long.

ORGANIC PRODUCE

It may well be worth it to pay a little extra for organically grown food, since non-organically grown produce frequently carries pesticides, which are harmful to humans if consumed.

LACTIC BACILLI

Our intestines are equipped with a unique self-defense mechanism because they are in the front line of defense as the effects of food enter our body. E coli attached to food has one unique characteristic: it is weak against acid. Lactic bacilli break down sugar inside the body and cause lactic acid fermentation. Lactic acid then causes the PH level to decrease inside the intestines by increasing the acidity, and this, in turn, suppresses the proliferation of E coli.

Lactic bacilli also produce a material called organic acid which stimulates the walls of the intestines and urges the peristalsis movement of the digestive tract so that a bowel movement is facilitated.

We have come to understand how to activate the digestive tract hormones, and we can safely say that the health of our intestines depends predominantly upon lactic bacilli. The secret of keeping our intestines healthy is to keep good bacteria working and suppress bad bacteria. We can do this by keeping a sufficient level of good bacteria in our intestines.

MELATONIN

We have already discussed the importance of melatonin for our health, particularly its role in our sleep rhythms. What may be surprising is that melatonin can be found in a variety of foods, especially rice, corn, oats, kale, and ginger.

HEALTHY HABITS

There are three points that, in addition to the suggestions above, will help your body use nutrients most effectively. The first point is that you must eat three meals regularly. If you miss a meal and eat a larger meal later, your blood sugar level increases suddenly, which causes a large amount of insulin to be secreted. If this condition persists, you will be more likely to suffer from low blood sugar, which can trigger depression and other mood changes. Your body's functions will be disrupted if you regularly skip meals.

For children especially, eating between meals is not a good idea because it may deter the secretion of growth hormones. Normally when we eat, our blood sugar level begins to increase in about thirty minutes. During the rise of this blood sugar level, the secretion of growth hormones slows down tremendously. Not until about ninety minutes after the meal will your body return to a normal blood sugar level. If a child eats often during the evening hours, the secretion of growth hormones can be curtailed. The irregularity of meals is affecting the secretion of growth hormones among children today, as more and more children stay home alone while their parents are at work.

As discussed earlier, growth hormones will not secrete once sex hormones kick in. Lately we are seeing cases of osteoporosis among young people. This is an alarming trend that may be related to the complex working of various hormones.

The second point to remember in maximizing your body's use of nutrients is that you should eat slowly. When you feel pressured because you are in a hurry, your sympathetic nerve system is strained, your heart rate increases, and you will be in a condition of stress. When your brain detects that you are in a stressful condition, it will secrete CRH to counter the stress. As a result, CRH will suppress appetite. If you force yourself to eat, you may experience nausea or stomach pain.

People who need to go to work early in the morning tend to wake up and rush to the breakfast table or rush to work with only toast for breakfast. That kind of lifestyle does not benefit hormone functioning in one's body. The best way to handle this is to wake up at least forty minutes before leaving for work. Do some light exercise to build up an appetite and then have a good breakfast. A glass of mineral water also aids digestion, prompting the smooth peristalsis movement of the digestive organs.

The third point is to enjoy your meal. When you are upset, gastric juice, bile, and pancreatic juice will not be secreted properly, nor will the hormones that handle digestion. When you eat in a peaceful state, digestion improves, and the hormones that are secreted will energize you more.

With forethought, care, and a little planning, a proper diet can be an additional weapon to help fight aging and illness. Proper diet and supplementation will also help you maintain a youthful appearance. Good nutrition is an absolutely essential part of any antiaging regimen.

Intelligently planned diet and nutrition are some of science's most effective, least expensive, and simplest life extenders and disease fighters—and virtually risk-free. The real surprise is how many of us are not willing to make the commitment to good diet and nutrition. If you're guilty of neglecting these proven life extenders, start planning new dietary habits today.

CHAPTER 15

Brain Boosters

KEEPING THE BRAIN AS FIT AS THE BODY

With the recent discovery of the aging gene telomerase came the research showing that telomerase can be controlled by hormones. The possibility of hormone replacement therapy being able to extend maximum human lifespans to 125 years or more is now closer to reality than ever before.

If you use hormone replacement therapy to return your body to its youthful state, practice optimal nutrition, exercise regularly, and keep stress levels to a minimum, you should live a long, full, and healthy life. Your body will function better than the bodies of others your age, and physically you will be able to keep up with people much younger. Although these strategies in the war against aging will help keep you mentally fit, there are concerns that your brain may not quite keep up with your body. The concern is that the discrepancy between the rate of aging of the brain and the rate of aging of the body will be magnified, given that the brain already ages faster than the rest of the body. This is particularly true if you have a family history of Alzheimer's disease, Parkinson's disease, or other degenerative brain disease.

WHY THE BRAIN AGES FASTER

To understand this concern, we must understand the brain. It is the second largest organ in the body, second only to our skin. It is the largest organ in weight and, unlike the other organs in the body which typically have specific roles, the brain has varied functions. The brain is responsible for initiating movement, perception, sensation, vision, thinking, memory, smell, hearing, and many other tasks. In addition, it is constantly communicating both with other parts of the body and with other parts of the brain. It is a constant hive of oxygen-hungry activity that uses about 40 percent to 50 percent of the oxygen intake of each breath. It is no wonder that the oxygen-hungry brain is the organ that is most affected by oxidative stress, one of aging's most significant processes.

BRAIN BOOSTERS

Fortunately, medical science is on the brink of wider use of several new therapies that fight oxidative stress and promote maximum brain function in the golden years. You may have even heard the popular term *smart drugs* used for the various substances that researchers now know boost brain function. The term smart drugs, however, is a misnomer, because the substances that boost the brain are not all drugs. What many in the medical community also call *nootropics* (Greek for "enhancing the brain"), we shall call *brain boosters.*

Brain boosters come in several different forms. Some are drugs that require a doctor's prescription; some are nutrients such as vitamins and amino acids; some are common herbs that have been used for centuries by other cultures; and some are hormones. If you are currently involved in a vitamin and mineral regimen or hormone replacement therapy, you may be taking some of them already.

Brain boosters work in one or more of the following ways:

- By slowing down the degeneration or aging of the brain
- By repairing damaged brain cells
- By increasing blood flow to the brain, enhancing the functions of existing brain cells or helping repair damaged ones
- By increasing neurotransmitters and helping build new networks in the brain

Some of the aspects of mental function that brain boosters impact and improve include alertness, intelligence, memory, learning ability, response time, and energy levels.

UNIQUE TO YOU

Because each brain booster has its own way of improving brain function, some brain boosters work better for some people than others. Finding the unique combination best suited for your maximum mental acuity is something you should pursue with your doctor. Partly, this is because some brain boosters can only be obtained with a prescription. In addition, the kinds of brain boosters that do work for you give your doctor a good indication of how your brain is aging. Armed with that knowledge, there may be other brain boosters that your doctor can then suggest. Additionally, there may be drugs, herbs, hormones, or nutrients that you are already taking that may need to be adjusted so you do not duplicate your body's efforts in one area while neglecting it in another.

Based on research currently available, the substances described in the following pages are the brain boosters that the Palm Springs Life Extension Institute now recommends and makes available to our patients.

HORMONE BRAIN BOOSTERS

All hormones that decrease as we age have the potential to impact the brain and should be replaced. What keeps the body healthy and the heart pumping effectively will also help keep the brain better nourished. However, in its ability to keep the brain healthy, one hormone stands out above the rest.

Pregnenolone

Pregnenolone is a non-prescription hormone that you may already be taking. If you are, keep taking it. Research has shown that this hormone is found in higher concentrations in the brain than in any other organ of the body. Those amounts often decrease significantly with age.

Pregnenolone has long been ignored by the medical community because it appeared to have no independent function other than to break down into DHEA and progesterone (which in turn break down into other steroids including cortisol, aldosterone, estrogen, and testosterone). Today we know that apart from producing other hormones, pregnenolone also minimizes inflammation, repairs damaged brain and spinal cord cells, allows our bodies to deal with stress more effectively, and is a potent memory enhancer.

More than fifty years of research supports the improvements in mental power that pregnenolone recipients claim. In addition to heightened acuity, test subjects reported increased energy, decreased fatigue, and improved mood, memory, and ability to cope with stress. Physical test results supported the subjects' claims to be able to better cope with stress by showing markedly reduced seventeen-ketosteroid urinary excretion, a substance excreted in response to higher levels of stress.[138]

Pregnenolone has the greatest memory-enhancing effect and produces that effect at doses one hundred times lower than other memory-producing agents. Pregnenolone not only prevents impaired memory from declining further, it actually appears to restore it.

DHEA

The ability of DHEA to help reverse age-related loss of cognitive function has been consistently demonstrated by research with laboratory animals. Small amounts lessen amnesia and enhanced long-term memory in mice. Mice also remembered what they had learned more effectively, even when given DHEA after the learning process had already taken place.[139] Because research with mice appeared so promising, human studies were undertaken that confirmed the memory-enhancing power of DHEA. Studies showed that DHEA blood levels are lower in Alzheimer's disease patients and that DHEA can slow or eliminate the progress of the disease.[140]

VIP—The Brain-Gut Hormone

The nerve cells of the cerebrum are responsible for processing information and performing calculations. Computers use tiny electrons for information processing. The nerve cells, on the other hand, use an electric current generated by the ions such as sodium,

---

138 Pincus G, Hoagland H. "Effects of administered pregnenolone on fatiguing psychomotor performances." *J Aviat Med* 15:98–115, 1944.

139 Birkenhager-Gillesse HG, et al. "DHEAS in the oldest old, aged 85 and over." *Ann NY Acad Sci* 719:543–552, 1994.

140 Flood JF, et al. "DHEA and its sulfate enhance memory retention in mice." *Brain Res* 447(2):269–278, 1988.

potassium, or chlorine to do the task. The signals are transmitted almost instantaneously inside the nerve fibers.

The hormone responsible for this fast transmission of information is called vasoactive intestinal peptide, or VIP. This hormone was originally discovered in the intestines, but later we found that the same hormone is distributed in a large quantity in the brain cortex. This hormone that is common to both the brain and the intestines (gut) is also known as the *Brain-Gut hormone.*

VIP operates to enlarge the capillary of the digestive tract and functions similarly in the brain. As a result, the blood circulation inside the brain increases to activate the nerve cells, and thus, information is transmitted faster. Indirectly, this will translate as a better functioning of the brain as well as an increased capacity for computation. Another interesting fact we have discovered is that when we give VIP to a mouse, it will act as if it were given dopamine, a hormone that causes elation and vitality. The mouse will get excited and begin to run around vigorously.

It's reasonable to assume that this hormone will increase our information-processing capability and the excitement the hormones bring to us will become the source of our creativity.

NUTRIENT BRAIN BOOSTERS

Other significant brain boosters that you may already be taking include nutrient brain boosters. Herbal, vitamin, amino acid, and antioxidant brain boosters have so many cross-over functions that it is simpler just to call them all nutrients. Their role in the brain—and it's an important one—is to provide maximum nutrition, improved blood flow, and minimum oxidation.

First let's tackle vitamins. Once again, all vitamins have significant roles to play in keeping our bodies healthy, and when our bodies are healthier, so are our brains. That said, recent studies confirm that the most important of these in the brain boosters are the following.

Vitamins B1, B2, B6, and B12

B vitamins help make neurotransmitters and promote the cell's ability to fight off disease,[141] while low levels of B vitamins are associated with memory loss.[142] Oral absorption of these vitamins declines with age, when we need higher and higher doses to maintain optimal levels. Each day, you should be getting at least 25 mg of B1, 100 mg of B2, 100 mg of B6, and 500 mg of B12. According to researchers, if your B vitamins are low, you may not be able to absorb enough from your multivitamin supplement and will need help from your doctor.[143] (Adequate oral absorption of B12 is a particular problem, and at the Palm Springs Life Extension Institute, we often add it to our patients' HGH injections.)

Vitamin E

We recommend vitamin E for its potent antioxidant properties and because research shows that it can slow mental decline tremendously. In a research project that tracked patients for two years, death, institutionalization, loss of ability to perform basic daily activities, and progression to severe dementia were postponed

---

141 Lesourd B. "Nutrition and immunity in the elderly: modification of immune responses with nutritional treatment." *Am J Clin Nutr* 66(2):478S–484S, 1997.

142 Wahlin A, et al. "Measurement of folic acid and vitamin B12 in the elderly. Low serum levels result in worse memory." *Lakaertidningen* 94(23):2177–2182, 1997.

143 Stabler SP, et al. "Vitamin B12 deficiency in the elderly: current dilemmas." *Am J Clin Nutr* 66(4):741–749, 1997.

Russell R. "New views on RDAs for adults." *J Am Diet Assoc* 97(5):515–518, 1997.

an average of two hundred thirty days in Alzheimer's patients who took two thousand IU of vitamin E per day.[144]

Vitamin A and Beta-Carotene

Vitamin A is required for the growth and protection of all organs, including the brain. Beta-carotene is a safe way to get vitamin A and, in addition, is a powerful antioxidant. It is converted into vitamin A in the liver when your body needs it, making it a safe source of the vitamin. The antioxidant properties of beta-carotene are now legendary, but beta-carotene's effects on the aging brain are also becoming well known. A twenty-two-year study published in 1997 concluded that antioxidants play an important part in brain health, and that among people ages sixty-five and older, higher ascorbic acid and beta-carotene plasma levels are associated with better recall, recognition, and vocabulary.[145] Beta-carotene supplements are non-toxic, even when taken in high doses.

COENZYME Q-10

CoQ10, or ubiquinone, is a vitamin-like compound that is necessary for energy production on a cellular level. The extra energy it brings to the cells of the immune system revitalizes the cells so they can do a better job of defending our bodies and our brains. It is a potent antioxidant that helps prevent the accumulation of free radical damage that can lead to degenerative diseases, particularly in the brain and heart. When CoQ10 levels drop with age, so does our general state of health. Low levels result in many health problems,

---

144 Sano M, et al. "A controlled trial of selegiline, alpha-tocopherol, or both as treatment for Alzheimer's disease." *New Engl J Med* 336(17):1216–1222, 1977.

145 Perrig WJ, Perrig P, Stahelin HB. "The relation between antioxidants and memory performance in the old and very old." *J Am Geriatr Soc* 45(6):718–724, 1997.

including high blood pressure, heart attacks, angina, immune system depression, gum disease, lack of energy, and obesity.

Many of these conditions impact brain health in a variety of ways. In a 1994 study of 113 psychiatric patients, high levels of CoQ10 deficiency were observed. After supplementation with CoQ10, many patients' conditions improved, none became worse, and none suffered any side effects.[146] Adding this potent antioxidant to our brain boosting arsenal could impact brain health at the cellular level.

Amino Acids

A complete complement of amino acids is another essential to a healthy brain. Amino acids are the building blocks or raw materials that the brain uses to make neurotransmitters. Amino acids are essential for all cell health. It is vital that you are ingesting enough of them if you are concerned about the maximum health of your body and your brain.

Acetyl-L-Carnitine

Acetyl-L-carnitine, or ALC, is another potent brain booster that is also considered a nutrient. It seems to work by improving blood flow to the brain and possibly enhancing the activity of the neurotransmitter acetylcholine. It is also believed to increase the number of neurotransmitters in the brain and to help promote recovery of the brain after a stroke or other brain damage. ALC also has the unique ability to destroy aging spots in the brain. We make this substance naturally, so it is a safe brain booster.

ALC has been well studied. It has been reported to improve motor skills, reflex time, and endurance, and to increase immunity,

146 Mesones HL. "Coenzyme Q-10 in psychiatry." *Acta Psiquiatr Psicol Am Lat* 40(3):207–210, 1994.

alertness, learning, memory, mood, and attention span, and to alleviate depression. Double-blind, placebo-controlled studies like those conducted in Italy by Alberto Spagnoli, MD, confirm these claims. Spagnoli reported that the drug slowed cognitive decline in patients with Alzheimer's disease. In fact, patients had significantly better results than untreated Alzheimer's patients in thirteen out of fourteen measures of mental functioning, including memory, attention, verbal capacity, and daily-living activities.[147] In June 1997, new animal studies were reported showing that rats given ALC after having suffered strokes recovered much more brain function than those of the control group.[148]

Choline and Lecithin

Choline and lecithin are the precursors of acetylcholine. They function in the brain by building neurotransmitters. They are especially important for vegetarians who may not get enough essential amino acids to keep neurotransmitter production at high levels.

Ginkgo Biloba

Ginkgo biloba is a an herb that has been used medicinally for centuries. It comes from a tree that itself often lives to be over one hundred years old. Ginkgo biloba is the only herb that has been through extensive clinical trials, and the only one that we currently recommend to our patients for brain boosting.

Ginkgo biloba has two important functions for brain boosting: it is a powerful antioxidant, and it improves circulation.

---

147 Spagnoli A, et al. "Long-term acetyl-L-carnitine treatment in Alzheimer's disease." *Neurology* 41(11):1726–1732, 1991.

148 Lolic MM, et al. "Neuroprotective effects of acetyl-L-carnitine after stroke in rats." *Ann Emer Med* 29(6):758–765, 1997.

DMAE (Dimethyl Amino Ethanol) and Centrophenoxine

In the United States, DMAE is a nonprescription health food substance. However, the European drug centrophenoxine, which breaks down to DMAE, is a prescription drug. DMAE has been reported to increase intelligence, memory, and learning ability.

We do not recommend DMAE, however. Patients develop a tolerance to DMAE, and so it is needed in larger and larger amounts to produce the same results. If the dose is increased above a certain level, side effects such as high blood pressure, insomnia, and headaches have been reported.

DRUG BRAIN BOOSTERS

Phosphatidylserine or PS

Phosphatidylserine, or PS, is another substance that appears to be useful in brain-function enhancement. PS is a component of the brain cell membranes and exists naturally in the body. It acts almost like a biological detergent, keeping fatty substances water soluble and thereby keeping cell membranes fluid and healthy. It helps the brain metabolize glucose more efficiently, builds new, healthier networks in the brain, and encourages the optimal functioning of existing brain cells.

In studies conducted in association with Stanford and Vanderbilt Universities, researchers gave 149 subjects PS three times a day for a period of twelve weeks. Tests performed before and after the clinical trial showed that those taking the PS rolled back the cognitive age clock by roughly twelve years.[149]

---

149 Crook TH, et al. "Effects of phosphatidylserine in age-associated memory impairment." *Neurology* 41:644–649, 1991.

Crook TH, et al. "Effects of phosphatidylserine in Alzheimer's disease." *Psychopharmacol Bull* 28:61–66, 1992.

In a 1988 Italian trial in which scientists gave phosphatidylserine to seventy Alzheimer's patients for three months, the researchers found that memory improved in all patients, and the improvement was maintained three months after the drug was withdrawn.[150] The results all suggest that phosphatidylserine may be a promising candidate for treating memory loss.

Deprenyl

Deprenyl, also known as selegiline, slows down production of monoamine oxidase-B (MAO), a natural but sometimes overly produced substance which at higher levels has been implicated in brain aging and Parkinson's disease. In addition to being the safest of the MAO inhibitors, deprenyl also increases the availability of the neurotransmitters dopamine, norepinephrine, and phenylethylamine, which play critical roles in motor, behavior, and cognitive functions. In animal studies, deprenyl improved memory, boosted cognitive function, increased lifespan by an amazing 40%, and consistently caused elderly rats to retain sexual vigor long past the age of untreated animals.[151] In more recent studies, patients with Parkinson's disease treated with L-dopa and deprenyl live significantly longer and more productively than those on L-dopa alone. And when taken by Alzheimer's patients, deprenyl significantly improves their condition.[152]

---

150 Amaducci L, and SMID group. "Phosphatidylserine in the treatment of Alzheimer's disease: results of a multicenter study." *Psychopharmacol Bull* 24(1):130–134, 1988.

151 Knoll J. "The striatal dopamine dependency of life span in male rats. Longevity study with (-) deprenyl." *Mech Ageing Dev* 46(1–3):237–262, 1988.

152 Knoll J. "The pharmacological basis of the beneficial effects of deprenyl in Parkinson's and Alzheimer's diseases." *J Neural Transm Suppl* 40:69–91, 1993.

People have been warned that deprenyl may have side effects, consisting of hot flashes and palpitations, if combined with cheese or wine, but this is highly unlikely. The much larger doses taken for Parkinson's disease are more likely to cause this kind of problem. If these symptoms occur after taking deprenyl, they are not dangerous, do not require emergency room treatment, and are best handled by sleeping them off.

Piracetam

Piracetam is a drug that is especially useful for stroke patients or those who have suffered any type of physical damage to the brain. This drug increases communication between the two halves of the brain. No other brain booster can do this.

Brain functions are often seated in particular areas of the brain. When that area is damaged, if the two halves of the brain are communicating well, other areas of the brain will, over time, assume the function of the damaged area. Piracetam is unequalled in aiding this process. According to United States law, individuals can buy a three-month supply of drugs for their own use from a country where that drug is legal. Most compounding pharmacies can put you in touch with off-shore, mail-order pharmacies where important drugs like piracetam can be obtained.

Hydergine

Hydergine is a drug that was formerly used for the treatment of high blood pressure. Patients being treated with this drug found their moods, memories, and congnition improved so much that researchers began to consider using it to treat Alzheimer's disease.

Hydergine has a wide range of brain-enhancing properties including: increasing the blood, and thereby oxygen, flow to the brain; enhancing the brain's ability to use the oxygen it receives; powerful antioxidant properties; protecting the brain from damage during periods of limited oxygen supply (such as after a stroke); and raising serotonin levels in the brain.

Hydergine also has a property unique to brain boosters in that it has the ability to aid protein synthesis and help regrow nerve connections and neurons, all of which help the brain regeneration now known to be possible. A variety of new nerve growth factors are currently being studied, but none have been approved for clinical use yet. This makes hydergine the only drug that can currently be taken to promote nerve growth.

BE ALL YOU WANT TO BE

If you are interested in taking all of these brain boosting substances in one convenient form, Palm Springs Life Extension Institute has created a brain booster capsule which contains hydergine, Ginkgo biloba, acetyl-L-camitine, coQ10, and phosphatidylserine. A brain booster capsule, taken with a high quality multiple vitamin-and-mineral supplement and amino acids, should help you achieve total brain boosting coverage.

DAILY HABITS TO BENEFIT YOUR BRAIN

If your hormones are optimized, your IQ will actually increase. You would be amazed what hormones can do for you in enhancing your abilities in the areas of memorization, creativity, and motivation. In order for your mind to be sharp, you must learn to activate the "Three S's" of hormone optimizing: sleep, sunshine, and symphonic music. Discover a "new you" as you allow the proper hormones to secrete abundantly in your body.

IQ has been used to measure intelligence for many years. It has been a belief that one's IQ is determined genetically, but this

IQ myth has been broken with an interesting experiment that involved studying and comparing the IQs of identical twins. The study clearly showed that identical twins with an identical genetic makeup develop a significant difference in IQ depending upon their educational environment. Through this study, we have now come to believe that almost 60 percent of one's IQ is determined by external factors. These external factors, such as education and environment, can either lower or raise one's IQ depending on the circumstances.

For example, it has been found that doing something as simple as changing the time of studying can raise one's memory. We knew that the ability to memorize resides in the area of our brain called the hippocampus, and the temporal lobe of the brain also has a role in memorization. Now we have discovered an important role hormones play in memorization. For example, ACTH (adrenocorticotropic hormone) especially improves short-term memory. When you need to memorize something, ACTH is triggered and secreted to allow your brain to concentrate on memorization. ACTH is secreted the most between 4:00 a.m. and 9:00 a.m. This time bracket is a golden time for memorization. If you sit at your desk during these hours to study or work, you will be amazed at the improvement in your mental acuity. If you measure the total amount of secretion during this time, you will discover that ACTH is secreted twice as much as it is during the rest of the night. If I was a student again and studying for an exam, I would opt to study in the early morning to utilize the full benefits of ACTH.

Vasopressin

Vasopressin is a hormone that improves long-term memory. Vasopressin secretes in an inverse proportion to the amount of water our body holds. If the amount of water in the body decreases by 1 percent, the amount of vasopressin increases twice as much. If the water increases by 1 percent, the vasopressin decreases twice as much. This is because this particular hormone detects the amount of water in the body and attempts to supply the water through re-absorption.

The human body is 70 percent water. If you weigh 60 kg, 42 kg of your weight is water. One percent of that water volume is 420 grams. Therefore, if you drink two cans of cola, the amount of vasopressin is decreased by exactly half. While you work or study, if you keep drinking cola, tea, or coffee, you are endangering the secretion of vasopressin to the point of lowering your memorization ability.

A Hot Bath

Bathing is another way to activate vasopressin so that your memorization skills heighten. When you get in a warm bath, you relax and feel good; however, the real benefit of bathing is the secretion of vasopressin. If you have to study at night, take a warm bath and then study.

Another hormone that will secrete when you bathe is cortisol. If you take a warm bath at 108° F at 9:00 p.m., the amount of cortisol secreted in your adrenal cortex will increase tremendously. If you go to sleep right away, cortisol will allow you to rest well during the night, and you will feel refreshed in the morning.

Many people have tried a cold bath in the early morning, the benefit of which can be substantiated, as cortisol will secrete more. Buddhist monks' disciplines included taking a cold bath in the early morning, which may have helped them have more cortisol in their systems. Thus, a cold bath in the early morning will enable you to be more productive at work.

Dopamine

We already discussed the neurotransmitter dopamine and its role in creative expression. The endocrinal gland of dopamine is distributed widely in the area of the brain cortex called the *association area*, which is responsible for our mental activities. The A10 nerve, which is located here, can send out a large amount of dopamine. In order to enhance creativity, we need to activate this A10 nerve so that more dopamine is secreted.

You can activate the A10 area by trying to remove anxiety from your mind and avoiding an unpleasant work environment that produces stress. Before you engage in any creative work, think about things that are happy or joyful. Give yourself generous compliments.

Early in the morning in a quiet place, meditate on positive thoughts. Your "A system" nerves will then become activated, and dopamine will be secreted in a large quantity. You will begin your day in a creative frame of mind.

CHAPTER 16

The Future

THE QUEST FOR LONGEVITY

Throughout the course of human history, there has been an ongoing but ever-elusive quest to lengthen the human lifespan. We are now closer than we have ever been. In recent years, scientists have provided us with indisputable evidence that caloric restriction, manipulation of telomerase, hormone replacement therapy, antioxidants, exercise, and avoiding stress, tobacco, environmental chemicals and toxins, pesticides, heavy metals, and ultraviolet rays, among other things, can change the course of age-related diseases and extend the human lifespan. Used in combination, these antiaging and longevity therapies can keep us younger than people our age have ever been. Right now, staying young is especially vital because the next ten years may yet prove to be the most important years of our lives!

THE BRIDGE YEARS

Why are the next ten years so important? Because they are the bridge years, the years when, if you can remain alive and healthy, antiaging and longevity medical knowledge will continue to grow exponentially, just in time for you to make use of it. If you can remain young and vital during the next ten years, who knows how far antiaging and longevity science will take us?

RESEARCH AVENUES

Antiaging and longevity research is currently so exciting that it's almost overwhelming. Longevity-related discoveries are being made every day in fields as diverse as stem cells, nutrition, genetic and telomeric research, and endocrinology. With each new discovery, we are one step closer to a maximum lifespan of one hundred twenty years, as in biblical times.

Make Hormone Levels Part of Your Annual Check-up

Someday it may become the standard of preventative medicine to begin testing twenty-year-olds for hormone deficiencies, so everyone can begin to guard their health by preventing any decline in hormone levels. But until that happens, millions of people will be exposed to years of lowered immunity and weakening bones and organs caused by dropping levels of certain hormones. Unfortunately, these people may not realize they have a hormone deficiency until something goes seriously wrong. We have already seen the tremendous power of hormone therapy (especially growth hormone treatment) in reversing and repairing damage caused by low hormone levels.

Why Some Diseases and Not Others?

We have already been delighted and surprised by the fact that hormones can effectively treat many common age-related diseases and illnesses. But certain conditions, such as congenital diseases like cystic fibrosis, cannot be treated by hormone therapy. Some of this may be because these diseases are caused by defective genes that require genetic therapy and have nothing to do with hormone deficiencies.

Scientists predict that our knowledge of antiaging medicine will grow at an exponential rate, increasing tenfold by the first decade of the twenty-first century. We may now be on the threshold of learning how to prevent and treat some or most of the devastating illnesses that affect millions of people.

While hormone therapy may never cure all illnesses, the potential for using hormone therapy to improve the quality of life is tremendous. One dramatic case in point is the effect that growth hormone has on HIV-positive and AIDS-infected individuals. Treatment with recombinant human growth hormone is not able to rid the body of the deadly virus, but it has been shown to delay the onset of full-blown AIDS and to greatly improve the quality of life for AIDS sufferers by increasing their bone and muscle strength and boosting the immune system.[153] There may be other diseases for which hormone therapy has a similar application. While we may not yet have the cures for certain conditions, proper hormone treatment can add healthy years to anyone's life.

---

153 Windisch PA, Papatheofanis FJ, Matuszewski KA. "Recombinant human growth hormone for AIDS-associated wasting." *Ann Pharmacother* 32(4):437–445, 1998.

Schambelan M, Mulligan K, Grunfeld C, et al. "Recombinant human growth hormone in patients with HIV-associated wasting. A randomized, placebo-controlled trial. Serostim Study Group." *Ann Intern Med* 125(11):873–882, 1996.

Building Better Hormone Delivery Systems

In addition to finding better answers for the above questions, hormone therapy research will almost certainly focus on better ways of administering the hormones. For example, testosterone administration has greatly improved over the past few years. Previously, this hormone was only available by injection. But now researchers have developed both gels and patches that make administration both more convenient and more physiologic.

It is reasonable to believe growth hormone administration will also improve, though improvements in HGH administration will probably be different from those found for testosterone. Earlier in the book, we explained some of the difficulties involved in HGH administration. The HGH molecule is too large to be absorbed using the methods that work for testosterone, such as the gel or patch. In July of 1996, a study was published documenting the effects of a sustained-release form of human growth hormone. Researchers gave a single injection of microspheres to monkeys. From this one injection, serum levels of recombinant HGH and insulin-like growth factor-1 (IGF-1) were elevated for more than a month. In fact, IGF-1 levels were higher than those traditionally seen in daily administration of the hormone. Methods of stabilization and encapsulation still have to be perfected before this method will be ready for human use, but it points to a future of promising new developments.[154]

---

154 Johnson OL, Cleland JL, Lee HJ, Charnis M, et al. "A month-long effect from a single injection of microencapsulated human growth hormone." *Nat Med* 2(7):795–799, 1996.

Johnson OL, Jaworowicz W, Cleland JL, et al. "The stabilization and encapsulation of human growth hormone into biodegradable microspheres." *Pharm Res* 14(6):730–735, Jun 1997.

Needle-free HGH

Many people still don't like the idea of a needle, no matter how infrequent injections may be. A company in southern California is currently developing an alternative to injection. The procedure involves inserting a package of powdered hormone into a plastic tube. One mechanism punctures the pouch, and then a squeeze of the trigger fills the chamber with a fine white powder that can be inhaled in one breath. The hormones would travel directly to the lungs, where they could be quickly and safely absorbed into the bloodstream. It is possible that this device, and other simpler methods of administering HGH, could be available in as little as five years.

OTHER HORMONE RESEARCH

Manufacturers and health care professionals are constantly coming up with new and improved administration for various hormones. Likewise, we are continually learning how all the hormones work together, and finding other substances that may stimulate healthy, physiologic releases of HGH, sex hormones, melatonin, thyroid, DHEA, and other hormones. Some current studies are focusing on the hormones we may not know as much about, such as insulin growth factor, nerve growth factor, and interleukins. Remember that it was only a few short years ago that human growth hormone was thought to be necessary only for HGH-deficient children during puberty.

IGF-1 treatment has proven effective in stimulating protein metabolism and immunity-enhancing lymphocytes, and in decreasing body fat. Low doses of IGF-1 also appear to be very well tolerated.[155] IGF-1 has received some less-than-positive press recently because increased IGF-1 levels have been found in some types of cancer. But it simply doesn't make sense to equate IGF-1 with cancer. Like HGH and telomerase, IGF-1 levels decline with age, at the same time that cancer rates rise. If IGF-1 had any direct connection to cancer, levels of cancer would decline with age as IGF-1 levels do.

From hormones to telomeres, our elusive quest to lengthen the human lifespan is closer now than ever before. Researchers from a hundred different disciplines are working on their small but significant parts of the antiaging and longevity puzzle, often oblivious to the work of others in related fields. We already have enough research to recommend the antiaging therapies of caloric restriction, antioxidant therapy, and exercise. In addition, if you stop smoking, avoid stress, and protect your skin from the sun,

---

155 Bianda T, Glatz Y, Bouillon R, et al. "Effects of short-term insulin-like growth factor-1 (IGF-1) or growth hormone (GH) treatment on bone metabolism and on production of 1,25-dihydroxycholecalciferol in GH-deficient adults." *J Clin Endocrinol Metab* 83(1):81–87, 1998.

Ghiron LJ, Thompson JL, Holloway L, et al. "Effects of recombinant insulin-like growth factor-1 and growth hormone on bone turnover in elderly women." *J Bone Miner Res* 10(12):1844–1852, 1995.

Sandstrom R, Svanberg E, Hyltander A, et al. "The effect of recombinant human IGF-1 on protein metabolism in post-operative patients without nutrition compared to effects in experimental animals." *Eur J Clin Invest* 25(10):784–792, 1995.

Gluckman P, Klempt N, Guan J, et al. "A role for IGF-1 in the rescue of CNS neurons following hypoxic-ischemic injury." *Biochem Biophys Res Commun* 182(2):593–599, 1992.

Grinspoon SK, Baum HB, Peterson S, et al. "Effects of rhIGF-1 administration on bone turnover during short-term fasting." *J Clin Invest* 96(2):900–906, 1995.

Jardieu P, Clark R, Mortensen D, Dorshkind K. "In vivo administration of insulin-like growth factor-1 stimulates primary B lymphopoiesis and enhances lymphocyte recovery after bone marrow transplantation." *J Immunol* 152(9):4320–4327, 1994.

these practices and health principles will help change the course of the age-related diseases that nature had planned for you.

If you choose hormone gene therapy to improve the quality of your life and to help extend your life, then you'll be doing as much as we know how to do right now to keep those telomeres long and healthy!

And as time goes by, if other significant and safe antiaging research comes to light, you can be sure you'll hear it from us first.

VICTORY DAY

The trend in medicine is to quantify results with a lot of numbers. In talking about antiaging, the impulse is to define success by the number of years a person can live. Extending chronological age is an important and exciting aspect of antiaging medicine, but more important than the lists of studies and numbers presented in some scientific journal is the individual victory that each person can experience with the return of health and vitality.

The V-day we're talking about will not be remembered with a downtown parade and celebrations in the street. Instead, it is a V-day that will be celebrated every morning when you get out of bed with energy and enthusiasm for the day. Every day you are strong, mentally healthy, and can participate in the activities you love, you win a great victory in the war against aging.

The miracle of hormone replacement has made these quiet victories possible, and you can experience them firsthand, today. As levels of technology and understanding increase, and more antiaging treatments become available, these victories—our personal V-days—will be even greater and more frequent.

But the first step is one each of us has to take on our own, regardless of the advances of technology. We each have to decide to fight the war into which we have been drafted. We have to use the knowledge we have been given, and that which is yet to come, to beat back the forces of aging. To do this, we must first accept the fact that aging is a disease that can be treated. As with any other war, knowing the enemy is the key to winning the battle. We have learned what causes the disease of aging and how it manifests itself in our bodies. With this knowledge, we can medically anticipate the enemy's next move and, in this way, gain the upper hand against the forces we contend with.

We can then take the process one step further and create new definitions for terms like *old age* and the *golden years*. (Hopefully, in the near future the term *old age* itself will be out of date.) The golden years no longer have to be the ones in which you are basking in the sunset of life, waiting for the final light to go out. Instead, the golden years can be those when you have the time, energy, drive, and wisdom to live life as you've always desired. These years can be the best you've ever experienced.

Unfortunately, most people are unaware of the strategic advantage we now have in the war against aging. Most people still dread the advancing years because of the physical and mental disabilities that have, until now, been inevitable. Anyone who has cared for an aging family member or friend knows the pain and agony the ailing individual suffers, and many of us have personally experienced the burden and fatigue of providing care.

Each year, the number of people over age seventy increases, and with the baby-boomer generation getting older, the population of older individuals will skyrocket. The economic and physical burden this will place on family members and the whole of society will be enormous. Frankly, current gerontological philosophies and medical practices will do little to alleviate the problems that loom. Treating every individual illness or ailment that comes along, and not taking significant action until problems become life threatening, will be like trying to save the *Titanic* by bailing water with a thimble. It won't work. We must find other solutions.

Since treatment itself is insufficient, we must do what we can to *prevent* health problems. Until scientists find a practical way to use the immortalizing enzyme telomerase, we can help ward off the disease of aging with health-conserving practices such as caloric restriction and antioxidant therapy. We can also improve our lifestyle, including our activity level, the food we eat, and whether or not we smoke or drink alcohol. But most importantly, we can help keep our telomeres as young as possible by using a balanced, full-spectrum hormone gene therapy. By replacing and rejuvenating the natural substances that have declined over the years, we can make the constant visits to the doctor, medicine chests full of daily doses of antibiotics, painful surgeries, lengthy hospital stays, and physical and mental disabilities things of the past. Old age, as we now know it, could become obsolete.

This technology is available now; you can take advantage of it today. We're excited about what the research has shown, and we're eagerly working to unveil the future of antiaging medicine. Most importantly, we wish to instill in you a sense of hope and optimism for the future. We want to give you the knowledge and, most importantly, the will to fight. We want you to plan a retirement account that will financially support your active lifestyle well into your hundreds.

We invite you to join the antiaging crusade and use the breakthroughs that have been laid at your feet to go on the offensive in this war. It is no longer a losing battle. We have been given the tools and the weapons to win. Now we issue the call to arms. There is no way to prevent the calendar from marching on, and we can't keep the birthdays from coming. But we can look forward to each birthday as a joyful celebration of living life to its fullest. We can help make the wish "and many more" actually meaningful. Each time you mark the passing of another year, it can be your own personal victory celebration—a celebration of long life, good health, and happiness.

The number of people living in Japan and America to advanced old age is already on the rise. There are some 5.7 million Americans age 85 and older, amounting to 1.8% of the population, according the the recent United States Census Bureau. That is projected to rise to 19 million, or 4.3%, by 2050 based on current trends. The percentage of Americans 100 and older is projected to rise to 600,00 centenarians.

Many scientists think that this is just the beginning. They are working on new ways to replace worn-out organs –and even to help the body rebuild itself with such new technology as transplanting of autologous Stem Cells.

It is important to understand that their aim is not just to increase the quantity of life its quality as well. A life span of 120 years seem well within reach in the near future with most of those years being vital and productive.

The Wake Forest Institute for Regenerative Medicine, led by Dr. Anthony Atala, has successfully grown bladders in a lab and implant them in children and teenagers suffering from congenital defects. The basic structure of the bladders was built using biodegradable materials and was then populated with stem cells from the patient (called autologous stem cell transplant) so their bodies would not reject the transplant. The Institute is now working to grow more than 30 different organs and tissues, including liver, bone and hearts.

At the McGowan Institute for Regenerative Medicine at the University of Pittsburgh, Dr. Stephen Badylak and his team is working with "extracellular matrix" – the material that gives structure to tissue-from pig bladders (known as the ECM technology). Dr. Badylak has used ECM to grow back the tips of patient's fingers that have been accidentally snipped off, and his colleagues have used it to cure early stage esophageal cancer by removing the cancerous portion and replacing that with ECM. The ECM cannot yet grow back entire limb, but the results so far are impressive.

Living longer would also mean both making and spending money longer. Most of us already do not expect to retire at 60s. People who live to 120 will use their additional years for second and third careers.

All these technologies, including hormone supplementation, provide a longer span of healthy years that will lead to greater wealth and prospects for happiness.

The idea of anti-aging/longevity medicine has its critics. But, I think arguments against health span and life span extension are often simply an appeal to the status quo. Everything that we have, socially and as individual, is based on richness of life. There can be no more basic obligation than to help ourselves and future generations to enjoy longer and healthier spans on the Earth that we share.

AUTHOR'S NOTE

As with anything new, it takes time before ideas are accepted. The whole field of antiaging medicine is still young, and there is still much to be learned. But we have come a long way in a very few years, and much of this is due to the efforts of Dr. Ronald M. Klatz. Dr. Klatz was fundamental in organizing the American Academy of Antiaging (A4M), founded in 1993, and he now serves as the president of that organization.

Changing perceptions is the first step to getting any new idea accepted. Dr. Klatz has worked to change the perception that aging is an inevitable part of life that should be accepted "gracefully." He has sought to get people to view aging as they do any other disease—as a health problem that, with the right treatment, can be overcome.

ABOUT THE AUTHOR

Dr. Edmund Chein practices in Palm Springs, California, and is regarded by many as one of the founding fathers of longevity and antiaging medicine. Dr. Chein received his training at the University of Southern California Los Angeles County Medical Center in Rehabilitation Medicine. Dr. Chein learned the importance of hormone balancing during these rehabilitation years when, after replacing hormones in patients with damaged glands, he could see tremendous differences in their recoveries.

In the early 1990s, Dr. Chein discovered that telomere found in the DNA controls human aging and that telomerase , which controls the length of the telomere, is in turn controlled by bio-identical hormones (not designer hormones). Dr. Chein parlayed this discovery into the Total Hormone Supplementation Therapy. He then collaborated a study with Dr. Cass Terry of the Medical College of Wisconsin, where they tested one thousand human subjects by replacing and balancing all the hormones in their bodies to optimal, youthful levels. The study showed that the method was safe, that human body systems and functions that deteriorate with age can be restored, and that Biological Age can be reversed. They also found that age-related conditions, such as elevated cholesterol, increased body fat, and decreased energy, stamina, immunity, and sexual function can all be eliminated. He subsequently renamed the treatment Telomerase Activating Therapy.

He was the first doctor in the United States to use Growth Hormone on adults clinically (not research), and to advocate balance of all bio-identical hormones that affect aging.

Dr. Chein holds patents for his discoveries in longevity and antiaging procedure in the United States, British Commonwealth, and the People's Republic of China.

In 1994, Dr. Chein founded the Palm Springs Life Extension Institute. Every year, the Institute is visited by hundreds of new patients who come from all over the world to visit the doctor who has the largest clinical base of patients in hormone replacement therapy and has now treated well over two thousand patients. Because of his expertise, Dr. Chein is in constant demand by the media and has appeared on numerous national television and radio shows. He has also appeared in a number of national publications, including *Newsweek, Gentleman's Quarterly, Marie Claire* magazine and *Der Spiegel* magazine in Germany.

In 1996, he founded the American Academy of Longevity Medicine so physicians and scientists could pursue and exchange ideas and information regarding this new specialty.

APPENDIX A

Determining Your Hormone Type

Before you can use hormones as your allies to good health, you must start by identifying your hormone type. The hormone type helps you identify your hormonal inclinations. Are you the type who can secrete dopamine without difficulty? Or do you have excess thyroid hormone? We have different personality types, body shapes, idiosyncrasies, and emotions, and hormones are responsible for these differences. We have termed such differences *hormone types*. Understanding your hormone type may preclude some of the illnesses or psychological disorders which may be more prevalent within certain hormone types.

The benefit is more than simply precluding certain disorders. You may actually be able to enjoy more memorization capability, mental concentration, and creativity. You may be able to develop characteristics that will attract others. Knowing your hormone type may therefore help you elevate your standard of a healthful life. It may be possible to lead a much more fulfilling life by consciously and carefully controlling the appropriate hormones.

Recently we have begun to pay closer attention to the *quality* of life rather than the mere *length* of life. In Japan, where the human lifespan is the longest in the world, it is imperative to search for a more meaningful life, especially in one's later years. Hormones are the key to unlocking the door to a more fulfilling life, even after we have surpassed the maximum life expectancy.

The classification of the hormone types will hopefully be useful for a further understanding of the hormones in the areas of developing human potential and intellect, prevention of aging, and preventive medicines.

THYROXIN CHECK

Let us begin by checking the various tendencies of your thyroid hormone. Thyroxin is particularly important among hormones; it is secreted more than others and provides the vitality that is so necessary for maintaining life. It controls metabolism and body temperature. When the thyroid hormone is not secreting properly, you will recognize many symptoms. You may be surprised to discover that these symptoms, while occurring all too often, are commonly overlooked.

When you notice any words that might apply to you, circle them. If you think it applies even a little, put a circle around it. Tally the scores. As a result, you will obtain numbers that are either positive (+) or negative (-). Use the reference chart on the bottom. If you have a positive (+) number, you may be experiencing an active thyroid. If the number is negative (-), your thyroid may be underactive. If the number is larger than 10, your thyroid is likely to be hyperactive. Illnesses that are likely to occur as a result of hyperactive or underactive thyroids are listed at the end of the book for your reference.

TEST 1

THYROID HORMONE CHECK

+ Degree of Hyperthyroidism

	Point
Eat a lot but do not gain weight	+2
Sweat a lot, and thirsty	+2
Strong heartbeat, hands tremble	+2
Thyroid glands are enlarged	+2
Instability of emotions	+3
Partial hair loss	+1
Outer eyebrows are thin	+1
Tend to have diarrhea	+2
Irregular or no menstruation	+2
Maximum blood pressure is high and minimum blood pressure is low	+2
Lack of concentration	-1
Lack of vitality	-2
Dry skin, lacking in resistance for cold weather	-1

Puffy	-3
Loss of hair	-3
Constipation	-2
Thickness of tongue	-2
Loss of memory, forgetfulness	-3
Anemic	-2
Excessive menstruation flow	-1
Total Score	

THYROID HORMONE CHECK REFERENCE CHART

+ Degree of Hyperthyroidism

From +15 to +20	Very possible
From +10 to +14	Possible
From +5 to +9	Suspicious
From +4 to -4	Not very likely
From -5 to -9	Suspicious
From -10 to -14	Possible
From -15 to -20	Very possible

- Degree of Hypothyroidism

If you score above +10 or below -10, you should consult your doctor right away.

ADRENOCORTICOTROPIC HORMONE CHECK

The adrenocorticotropic hormone is essential in maintaining homeostasis and fighting against various stresses, both physical and mental, to keep the body functioning. Fighting against stress is done in a series of cooperative plays starting with CRH (hypothalamus). It then moves on to ACTH (pituitary) and ends with the adrenaline and cortisol hormones (adrenal gland).

If CRH becomes excessive in the hypothalamus, you will experience insomnia, depression, and lack of appetite. If it becomes inactive in the brain cortex, Alzheimer's disease may develop. ACTH is closely linked to memory and the ability to concentrate. If there is too much cortisol, Cushing's disease or Addison's disease may develop. If the hormones secrete normally, you will have a good chance of fighting off stress. In this test, we want to see if there is an imbalance of adrenocorticotropic hormones. Tally the results the same way as before. If you score above 10 (either in plus or minus), you should do blood tests and/or see a hormone doctor for further evaluation.

TEST 2

ADRENOCORTICOTROPIC HORMONE CHECK

	Point
Overweight, especially in the stomach area	+3
Tend to have a lot of body hair	+2
Round face with skinny limbs	+3
Frequent headaches, dizziness, stiff neck	+2
High blood sugar count (diabetes)	+2
Loss of muscle strength	+2
Bones tend to break more often	+1
Frequent acne	+2
Athlete's foot	+1
Irregular menstruation or impotence	+2
Fatigue	-2
Loss of weight	-2
Nausea	-3
Lack of appetite	-1
Low blood pressure	-2

Low blood sugar level	-2
Loss of hair for females (armpit and pubic hair)	-3
Prone to anger	-1
Brown discoloration of skin	-2
Tendency for diarrhea	-2
Total Score	

ADRENOCORTICOTROPIC HORMONE CHECK REFERENCE CHART

+ Suggests Degree of Likelihood of Hyperactive Adrenal Function

From +15 to +20	Very possible
From +10 to +14	Possible
From +5 to +9	Suspicious
From +4 to -4	Not very likely
From -5 to -9	Suspicious
From -10 to -14	Possible
From -15 to -20	Very possible

- Suggests Degree of Likelihood of Low Adrenal Function

TEST 3

SEX HORMONE CHECK

The purpose of this test is to measure your femininity or masculinity. At the time of puberty, female and male traits develop as a result of sex hormone secretions. However, the male hormone is not limited to males, and the female hormone is not limited to females. Testosterone, the male hormone, and estrogen, the female hormone, can be traced back to the common root hormone called DHEA. You need sex hormones of the opposite sex. However, the imbalance of sex hormones can cause serious problems. There are two tests, one for males and the other for females.

FEMALE HORMONE CHECK
For Females Only

	Point
Smooth skin	+3
Not very tall, early menstruation start	+2
Full and glossy hair	+3
Well-developed breasts and hips	+3

Small amount of body hair (armpits and limbs)	+3
Wider waist	+3
Heavier than average	+3
Stability of emotions, gentle	+2
Prefers marriage to career	+2
Abundance of hair	-3
Coarse hair	-3
Small breasts, small hips	-2
Frequent acne, pimples	-2
Coarse skin	-2
Enlarged clitoris	-3
Tall and sturdy	-2
Late start of menstruation	-2
Little or no menstruation	-3
Fond of sports, athletic games	-2
Total Score	

REFERENCE CHART

FEMALE HORMONE LEVELS

Over +20	Satisfactory
From +15 to +20	Slightly lacking
From -10 to +14	Suggests possible deficiency of female hormones. Recommend blood level checkup.
Below -10	Recommend medical check plus female hormones to be measured.

MALE HORMONE CHECK
For Males Only

	Point
Muscular, tall, and sturdy	+3
Hair on chest, arms, and legs	+3
Thick beard	+3
Front head hair is thin	+2
Instability of emotions	+2
Body odor, sensitive nose	+2
Aggressive, desire to conquer	+3
Low and strong voice	+3
Strong sexual desire	+3
Tall and lanky	-3
Little body hair	-2
No protrusion of Adam's apple, no voice change	-3
Thin and soft hair	-3
Enlarged breast	-3
Prefers girl toys	-2
Mild manners, not prone to fight	-2
No strong sexual desires	-2
More fat than muscles	-2
Smooth skin	-3
Dislikes sports, athletic games	-2
Total Score	

REFERENCE CHART

MALE HORMONE LEVELS

Over +20	Satisfactory
From +15 to +20	Slightly lacking
From -10 to +14	Suggests possible deficiency Recommend blood level check-up
Below -10	Recommend medical check plus male hormones to be measured

Hormone type can be derived by multiplying your mind hormone by your body hormone. (For example, it will appear as d – n – s.)

MEN'S ANDROPAUSE AND WOMEN'S MENOPAUSE HORMONE CHECK

Shortly after women reach the age when menstruation ceases, they go through a difficult time called menopause. The onset of menopause is different among individuals. When a woman reaches her forties, she needs to be cautious and aware, because some hidden disorders may surface.

Andropause for men seems to come about gradually. More recently, it may be due to societal stresses and pressures; many men seem to go through fairly rapid changes once they reach around 45 years of age. In the past, men functioned as young men even in their 60s, with room to spare. Men seem to be more diverse in individual differences than women in this respect. Factors such as genes, diet, and attitudes can play important roles.

Following are two tests, one for men and the other for women.

MENOPAUSE CHECK FOR WOMEN

SYMPTOMS	FREQUENT	LITTLE	NONE
Headaches, dizziness, stiff neck	2	1	0
Declining sexual desire	2	1	0
Nails and bones seem brittle	3	2	0
Shallow sleep	3	2	0
Irregular periods	3	2	0
Heavier flow and fewer days	3	2	0
Weight Gain	3	2	0
Hot flashes, sweating more	4	2	0
Cold in legs and hands	4	2	0
Out of breath, fast heartbeat, irritable	4	2	0
Difficult sleeping	4	3	0
Loss of elasticity in skin	4	3	0
Infection in urinary tract, difficulty or frequency in urination	5	3	0
Curled pubic hair grows straight	5	3	0
Pain during intercourse	5	3	0
Incontinency	5	4	0
Loss of height	5	3	0
Total Scores			

Below 5	Not yet menopause
6 - 20	Early stage of menopause
21 - 30	Menopause in progress
31 - 40	Start considering hormone replacement supplementation for menopause
Above 41	Consider hormone replacement supplementation for menopause

ANDROPAUSE CHECK FOR MEN
(Sapporo Medical School Kumamoto modified checklist)

A. Declining Sexual Activities	Points
Lost interest in opposite sex? Lower sexual desire	3
No erection when you see stimulating pictures? Lower erection ability	3
Decreased frequency of sexual activities? Fewer number of sexual activities	3
Can you maintain an erection? Shorter duration	3
B. Mental Health	
Are you tired more often?	2
Have you been depressed more?	2
Any insomnia?	2
Do you feel more lethargic in the morning?	2
Are you experiencing loss of appetite? Do you find food tasteless sometimes?	1
Do you feel you are losing productivity at work? Do you feel it is bothersome to perform many jobs?	1
Do you find your life meaningless?	2
C. Physical Conditions	
Do you feel tingling or "coldness" in legs, arms, and lower back?	1
Do you feel numbness in your hands or feet?	1
Do you feel that your feet and hands are not as sensitive?	1
Do you have headaches?	1
Does you heart seem to beat harder?	1
Do you sometimes feel as if ants are crawling on your skin?	1
Do you feel out of breath and as if you may suffocate?	1
Do you feel as if you have something lodged in your throat?	1
Have you lost weight recently?	1

Do you feel that your muscles are weaker?	1
Constipation?	1
Increased fat in your body?	1
Total Score	

Below 5	Not yet andropause
6 - 10	Early stage of andropause
11 - 20	Start considering hormone replacement supplementation for andropause
Above 21	You must consider hormone replacement supplementation for andropause

APPENDIX B

~

Sample Prescription for Biological Age Tests

EDMUND CHEIN, MD, JD
2825 TAHQUITZ CANYON, BLDG. A
PALM SPRINGS, CA 92262
(619) 327-8939 FAX (619) 327-0844
CA LIC. NO. A38678

NAME: ____

ADDRESS: ____

DATE: __________________________

BIOLOGICAL AGE TESTS

RX

1) Forced Vital Capacity *(Lungs)*
2) Cardiac Function Test (stress/treadmill test and/or cardiac hemodynamic studies) *(Heart)*
3) Creatinine Clearance Test *(Kidneys)*
4) Bone Density Scan *(Bone)*
5) Memory Test and Reaction Time *(Nervous System)*
6) T-Cell Subset Blood Test (CD4, CD8, Total T-Cell, Total Natural Killer Cell Count) *(Immune System)*

____

Edmund Chein, MD

APPENDIX C

EDMUND Y. CHEIN, MD CA LIC #A38678 DEA #AC1643661
2825 TAHQUITZ WAY, BLDG.A
PALM SPRINGS, CA 92262
(760) 327-8939 FAX (760) 327-0844
TOLL FREE 800-230-2144

The following Hormone/Blood Test order can be performed at any local medical laboratory, in any state or country. Please call our office at (800) 230-2144 to set up an appointment for a blood draw. When you receive your lab report you may call the Palm Springs Life Extension Institute to speak with one of our medical personnel or set up an appointment. If you have already scheduled an appointment, we look forward to reviewing your results when you visit the clinic.

STATUS: ☐ NEW PATIENT ☐ EXISTING PATIENT DATE: ________________

NAME: ____________________
ADDRESS: ____________________
CITY: ____________________ STATE: __________ ZIP: ____________
PHONE: ____________________
FAX: ____________________
DATE OF BIRTH: ______________ APPT. DATE / TIME: ______________
LAB: ☒ **MALE**
PLEASE PERFORM ONLY TESTS MARKED AND GIVE COPY TO PATIENT
RX: BLOOD TEST TO BE DONE AROUND LUNCH (12:00 PM – 1:30 PM)

FULL PANEL:

- ☐ SERUM SOMATOMEDIN—C (IGF-1) *(To be drawn after 12:00 noon after a 12-hour fasting period)*
- ☐ IGF BINDING PROTEIN 3
- ☐ TOTAL AND FREE TESTOSTERONE
  - ☐ *If using Testosterone Gel, test to be drawn 5 hours after applying gel in the morning*
  - ☐ *If taking Testosterone Cypionate, test to be drawn 4–5 days after the shot*
- ☐ DHEA SULFATE
- ☐ FREE T3, TSH, FREE T4 *(Every 6 months)*
- ☐ PREGNENOLONE
- ☐ COMPLETE METABOLIC PANEL
- ☐ CBC
- ☐ LIPID PANEL, CHOLESTEROL, HDL, TRIGLYCERIDE *(After fasting for eight hours)*
- ☐ TWELVE-HOUR FASTING SERUM INSULIN LEVEL
- ☐ ULTRA FAST CAT SCAN OF CORONARY ARTERY
- ☐ DHT (dihydrotestosterone)
- ☐ PSA *(Should be done yearly)*
- ☐ PET SCAN

ADDITIONAL TESTS:

- ☐ 24-HOUR URINE V.M.A. AND METANEPHRINES TEST *(For obese patients only)*
- ☐ CORTISOL
- ☐ SERUM TRIGLYCERIDE *(After fasting for eight hours)*
- ☐ TOTAL CHOLESTEROL
- ☐ LIVER ENZYMES
- ☐ SERUM LH
- ☐ ACTH
- ☐ % FREE PSA
- ☐ PROLACTIN
- ☐ ESTRADIOL
- ☐ PROGESTERONE

______________________ ______________________

EDMUND Y. CHEIN, MD *DATE*

EDMUND Y. CHEIN, MD CA LIC #A38678 DEA #AC1643661
2825 TAHQUITZ WAY, BLDG.A
PALM SPRINGS, CA 92262
(760) 327-8939 FAX (760) 327-0844
TOLL FREE 800-230-2144

The following Hormone/Blood Test order can be performed at any local medical laboratory, in any state or country. Please call our office at (800) 230-2144 to set up an appointment for a blood draw. When you receive your lab report you may call the Palm Springs Life Extension Institute to speak with one of our medical personnel or set up an appointment. If you have already scheduled an appointment, we look forward to reviewing your results when you visit the clinic.

STATUS: ☐ NEW PATIENT ☐ EXISTING PATIENT DATE:

NAME: ____________________
ADDRESS: ____________________
CITY: ____________________ STATE: _____ ZIP: __________
PHONE: ____________________
FAX: ____________
DATE OF BIRTH: ____________ APPT. DATE / TIME: ____________
LAB: ☒ **FEMALE** *PLEASE PERFORM ONLY TESTS MARKED AND GIVE COPY TO PATIENT*
RX: BLOOD TEST TO BE DONE AROUND LUNCH (12:00 p.m. – 1:30 p.m.)

FULL PANEL:

☐ SERUM SOMATOMEDIN – C (IGF-1) *(To be drawn after 12:00 noon after a 12-hour fasting period)*
☐ IGF BINDING PROTEIN 3
  ☐ *Menstruating female patients to do this test on the 1st–10th day of menstrual cycle*
☐ TOTAL AND FREE TESTOSTERONE
  ☐ *If using Testosterone Gel, test to be drawn 5 hours after applying gel in the morning*
☐ DHEA SULFATE
☐ FREE T3, TSH, FREE T4 *(Every 6 months)*
☐ PREGNENOLONE
☐ COMPLETE METABOLIC PANEL
☐ CBC
☐ LIPID PANEL, CHOLESTEROL, HDL, TRIGLYCERIDE (8 hours FASTING)
☐ 12 HR. FASTING SERUM INSULIN LEVEL
☐ ESTRADIOL
☐ PROGESTERONE
☐ PET SCAN
☐ ULTRA FAST CAT SCAN OF CORONARY ARTERY

ADDITIONAL TESTS:

- ☐ 24-HOUR URINE V.M.A. AND METANEPHRINES TEST *(For obese patients only)*
- ☐ CORTISOL
- ☐ SERUM TRIGLYCERIDE *(After fasting for eight hours)*
- ☐ TOTAL CHOLESTEROL
- ☐ LIVER ENZYMES
- ☐ SERUM LH
- ☐ ACTH
- ☐ % FREE PSA
- ☐ PROLACTIN
- ☐ DHT (dihydrotestostrone)
- ☐ PSA *(Should be done yearly)*

______________________________ ____________________

EDMUND Y. CHEIN, MD *DATE*

APPENDIX D

0021-972X/01/$03.00/0
The Journal of Clinical Endocrinology & Metabolism

Vol. 86, No. 5
Printed in U.S.A.

A Randomized Controlled Trial of Low-Dose Recombinant Human Growth Hormone in the Treatment of Malnourished Elderly Medical Patients*

LEUNG-WING CHU, KAREN S. L. LAM, SIDNEY C. F. TAM, WAYNE J. H. C. HU, SAU-LAN HUI, ANNA CHIU, KA-CHUN CHIU, AND PAULINE NG

Divisions of Geriatric Medicine (L.-W.C., W.J.H.C.H., S.-L.H., K.-C.C.) and Endocrinology and Metabolism (K.S.L.L.), University Department of Medicine, Queen Mary Hospital, The University of Hong Kong, Hong Kong SAR, China; and Division of Clinical Biochemistry (S.C.F.T.) and Department of Dietetics (A.C., P.N.), Queen Mary Hospital, Hong Kong SAR, China

ABSTRACT

High-dose recombinant human GH (rhGH) has been shown to improve the nutritional status of malnourished older adults. It is uncertain whether low-dose rhGH is effective and whether its effect on nutritional status will lead to any improvement in physical function. There is also no data on the outcome after a short course of rhGH treatment. The objectives of this study were to determine the efficacy of low-dose rhGH treatment for 4 weeks in malnourished elderly patients, its effect on physical functions, and the intermediate term outcome after a 4-week rhGH treatment. The study design was a randomized, placebo-controlled, double-blind trial conducted in a university teaching hospital. The patients were 19 medically stable malnourished elderly subjects. Intervention in the rhGH group was as follows: rhGH (Saizen, Serono, Switzerland) 0.09 IU/kg body weight (BW) 3 times weekly were given together with appropriate dietary intervention as prescribed by the dietitian. In the placebo group, equal volumes of normal saline per kilogram BW were given 3 times weekly together with the dietary intervention.

The baseline demographic, anthropometric, nutritional, and hematological variables, measures of physical function, and insulin-like growth factor I levels in both groups were comparable. Compared with the placebo group, the GH-treated group showed a more rapid gain in BW (after 3 weeks, +1.27 ± 0.36 *vs.* −0.28 ± 0.37 kg; $P = 0.008$), total lean body mass (change after 3 weeks by bio-impedance analysis, +1.45 ± 0.36 *vs.* −0.37 ± 0.48 kg; $P = 0.009$) and a faster improvement in 5-m walking time (decrease after 4 weeks, 23.79 ± 9.41 *vs.* 0.45 ± 4.62 sec; $P = 0.047$). The hemoglobin level rose more in the rhGH than the placebo groups (change at 8 weeks, +0.84 ± 0.34 *vs.* −0.42 ± 0.29 g/dL; $P = 0.012$). Serum albumin level also showed a greater delayed increase in the rhGH group than in the placebo group (change at 8 weeks, +5.1 ± 0.8 *vs.* 1.6 ± 1.2 g/dL; $P = 0.023$). There was no statistically significant difference for other nutritional variables. There was a greater rise in the mean serum insulin-like growth factor I level at 4 weeks in the GH than in the placebo groups (197 ± 58 *vs.* 54 ± 26 U/L; $P = 0.034$). The improvement in the rhGH group gradually diminished on follow-up and became statistically insignificant 8 weeks after stopping rhGH treatment. There were no GH-related adverse effects.

Low-dose rhGH was an effective and safe adjuvant to dietary augmentation for stable malnourished elderly subjects. It led to a faster gain in total lean body mass, which was associated with greater improvement in walking speed when compared with dietary intervention alone. There were no apparent side effects. (*J Clin Endocrinol Metab* **86:** 1913–1920, 2001)

MALNUTRITION IS common in elderly people with chronic diseases. The prevalence of protein-energy under-nutrition in the elderly medical patients has been reported to be 17–44% (1–4). Undernourished elderly not only have an increased chance of mortality, but are at increased risk of impaired immune function, infections, impaired muscle function, falls, and deterioration of functional status (5–10).

Clinical management principally includes the treatment of the underlying cause and nutritional intervention. The standard treatment approach in nutritional repletion is by increasing the protein and energy intake in the diet, and nutritional supplementation has been shown to be an effective means of providing additional nutrients on top of the usual diet (11).

Aging is associated with decreased GH secretion and dynamic response (12). The beneficial effects of GH replacement in GH-deficient children and adults have been well reported (13). GH is a potent protein anabolic agent. Several studies of 1–3 weeks duration using moderate doses of recombinant human GH (rhGH) in postoperative subjects and malnourished elderly [rhGH 0.3 IU/kg body weight (BW) daily] have shown promising positive results in nitrogen balance and weight gain, with no accompanied adverse effect (14–16). Low-dose rhGH replacement (rhGH 0.09 IU/kg BW 3 times per week) for 6 months in healthy elderly men also improved body composition (17). However, side effects such as edema of the lower limbs, diffuse arthralgia, hand stiffness, gynecomastia, and carpal tunnel syndrome were common (17–21). These side effects subsided after the reduction of GH dose by 25–50% (17).

There are no published data on the efficacy of low-dose rhGH in the treatment of protein-energy malnourished elderly patients. It is uncertain whether any beneficial effect on

Received October 9, 2000. Revised December 28, 2000. Accepted January 29, 2001.

Address all correspondence and requests for reprints to: Dr. L. W. Chu, F.R.C.P. (Edinburgh and Glasgow), Division of Geriatric Medicine, University Department of Medicine, The University of Hong Kong, Queen Mary Hospital, 102 Pokfulam Road, Hong Kong SAR, China. E-mail: lwchu@hkucc.hku.hk.

* Part of the laboratory cost was sponsored by Serono Pharmaceuticals (Hong Kong) Ltd. (Hong Kong, China).

APPENDIX E

Date
January 5, 1999

Patent Number
5,855,920

Edmund Chein, M.D.

INVENTOR

TOTAL HORMONE REPLACEMENT THERAPY

The Director of the United States Patent and Trademark Office has received an application for a patent for a new and useful invention. The requirements of law have been complied with, and it has been determined that a patent on the invention shall be granted under the law.

Therefore, this

United States Patent

Grants to the person(s) having title to this patent the right to exclude others from making, using, offering for sale, or selling the invention throughout the United States of America or importing the invention into the United States of America for the term of this patent, subject to the payment of maintenance fees as provided by law.

Acting Commissioner of Patents and Trademarks

(12) UK Patent Application (19) GB (11) 2 320 190 (13) A

(43) Date of A Publication 17.06.1998

(21) Application No 9715349.8

(22) Date of Filing 21.07.1997

(30) Priority Data
(31) 08766320 (32) 13.12.1996 (33) US

(71) Applicant(s)
Edmund Y M Chein
Building A, 2825 Tahquitz Canyon Way, Palm Springs, California 92262, United States of America

(72) Inventor(s)
Edmund Y M Chein

(74) Agent and/or Address for Service
Abel & Imray
Northumberland House, 303-306 High Holborn, LONDON, WC1V 7LH, United Kingdom

(51) INT CL[6]
A61K 38/27 // (A61K 38/27 31:40 31:565 31:57 38:30 38:32)

(52) UK CL (Edition P)
A5B BJA B24Y B240 B45Y B450 B48Y B482 B55Y B551 B57Y B575 B61Y B616
U1S S2412 S2413

(56) Documents Cited
WO 95/32991 A1 US 4902680 A

(58) Field of Search
UK CL (Edition O) **A5B BJA BJB**
INT CL[6] **A61K 38/22 38/27**
ONLINE: CAPLUS, WPI, CLAIMS, JAPIO

(54) **Hormone replacement therapy involving human growth hormone (somatotropin)**

(57) There is described a multi-component hormone supplement therapy comprising human growth hormone (HGH/somatotropin) and at least two other hormones selected from a sex hormone, an adrenal hormone, a thyroid hormone, a thymic hormone or melatonin. Preferably the androgens are testosterone, oestrogen, pregnenolone, progesterone or dehydroepiandrosterone (DHEA). Insulin-like growth factor IGF-I is preferably also included. In the preferred method all of the aforementioned hormones are used.

GB 2 320 190 A

发明专利证书

证书号 第230202号

发明名称：全面性激素替代治疗法

发明人：爱德慕·全恩

专利号：ZL 98 1 01688.X　　国际专利主分类号：A61K 38/22

专利申请日：1998年4月30日

专利权人：爱德慕·全恩

授权公告日：2005年10月5日

本发明经过本局依照中华人民共和国专利法进行审查，决定授予专利权，颁发本证书并在专利登记簿上予以登记。专利权自授权公告之日起生效。

本专利的专利期限为二十年，自申请日起算。专利权人应当依照专利法及其实施细则规定缴纳年费。缴纳本专利年费的期限是每年04月30日前一个月内。未按照规定缴纳年费的，专利权自应当缴纳年费期满之日起终止。

专利证书记载专利权登记时的法律状况。专利权的转让、继承、撤销、无效、终止和专利权人的姓名、国籍、地址变更等事项记载在专利登记簿上。

专利号

局长 田力普

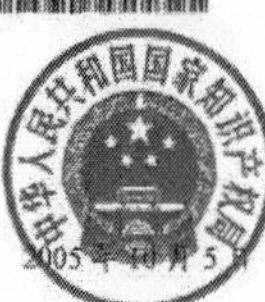

第1页（共1页）

BIBLIOGRAPHY

Adlercreutz CH, Goldin BR, Gorbach SL, Hockerstedt KA, Watanabe S, Hamalainen EK, Markkanen MH, Makela TH, Wahala KT (Department of Clinical Chemistry, Helsinki University Central Hospital, Finland.) "Soybean phytoestrogen intake and cancer risk." *J Nutr* 125(7):1960, Mar 1995.

Althaus BU, Staub JJ, Ryff-De Leche A, Oberhansli A, Stahelin HB. ~~(Department of Medicine, University Hospital, Basel, Switzerland.)~~ "LDL/HDL changes in subclinical hypothyroidism: possible risk factors for coronary heart disease." *Clin Endocrinol* 28:157–163, Feb 1988.

Amaducci L. "Phosphatidylserine in the treatment of Alzheimer's disease: results of a multicenter study." *Psychopharmacol Bull* 24(1):130–134, 1988.

Amato G, Izzo G, La Montagna G, Bellastella A. (Department of Endocrinology, Faculty of Medicine and Surgery, Second University of Naples, Italy.) "Low dose recombinant human growth hormone normalizes bone metabolism and cortical bone density and improves trabecular bone density in growth hormone deficient adults without causing adverse effects." *Clin Endocrinol (Oxf)* 45:27–32, Jul 1996.

Andreone P, Cursaro C, Gramenzi A, Zavagliz C, Rezakovic I, Altomare E, Severini R, Franzone JS, Albano O, Ideo G, Bernardi M, Gasbarrini G. (Patologia Medica 1, Universita di Bologna, Italy.) "A randomized controlled trial of thymosin-alpha 1 versus interferon alfa treatment in patients with hepatitis B e antigen antibody—and hepatitis B virus DNA—positive chronic hepatitis B." *Heptatology* 24(4):774–777, Oct 1996.

Arslanian SA, Becker DJ, Lee PA, Drash AL, Foley TP Jr. "Growth hormone therapy and tumor recurrence. Findings in children with brain neoplasms and hypopituitarism." *Am J Dis Child* 138(4):347–350, Apr 1985.

Arver S, Dobs AS, Meikle AW, Allen RP, Sanders SW, Mazer NA. (Department of Molecular Medicine, Karolinska Institute, Stockholm, Sweden.) "Improvement of sexual function in testosterone deficient men treated for one year with a permeation enhanced testosterone transdermal system." *J Urol* 155(5):1604–1608, May 1996.

Astrom C, Christensen L, Gjerris F, Trojaborg W. (Department of Clinical Neurophysiology, Rigshospitalet-University Hospital, Copenhagen, Denmark.) "Sleep in acromegaly before and after treatment with adenectomy." *Neuroendocrinology* 53:328–331, Apr 1992.

Astrom C, Lindholm J. (Department of Clinical Neurophysiology, University Hospital, Rigshospitalet, Copenhagen, Denmark.) "Growth hormone-deficient young adults have decreased deep sleep." *Neuroendocrinology* 51:82–84, Jan 1990.

Astrom C, Pedersen SA, Lindholm J. (Department of Clinical Neurophysiology, University Hospital, Copenhagen, Denmark.)

"The influence of growth hormone on sleep in adults with growth hormone deficiency." *Clin Endocrinol (Oxf)* 33:495–500, Oct 1990.

Bailey AR, Smith RG, Leng G. (Department of Physiology, University Medical School, Edinburgh, UK.) "The nonpeptide growth hormone secretagogue, MK-0677, activates hypothalamic arcuate nucleus neurons in vivo." *J Neuroendocrinol* 10(2):111–118, Feb 1998.

Ball SE, Gibson FM, Rizzo S, Tooze JA, Marsh JC, Gordon-Smith EC. (Division of Haematology, Department of Cellular and Molecular Sciences, St. George's Hospital Medical School, London, UK.) "Progressive telomere shortening in aplastic anemia." *Blood* 91(10):3582–3592, May 1998.

Barnes B. *Hypothyroidism: The Unsuspected Illness.* New York: Harper Collins, 1976.

Barrett-Connor E, Khaw KT, Yen SS. "A prospective study of dehydroepiandrosterone sulfate, mortality and cardiovascular disease." *N Eng J Med* 315(24):1519–1524, Dec 1986.

Beardsley T, Pierschbacher M, Wetzel GD, Hays EF. "Induction of T-cell maturation by a cloned line of thymic epithelium (TEPI)." *Proc Natl Acad Sci* 80:6005, Oct 1983.

Bengtsson BA, Eden S, Lonn L, Kvist H, Stokland A, Lindstedt G, Bosaeus I, Tolli J, Sjostrom L, Isaksson OG. (Department of Medicine, Sahlgrenska Hospital, Medical Faculty, University of Goteborg, Sweden.) "Treatment of adults with growth hormone (GH) deficiency with recombinant human growth hormone." *J Clin Endocrinol Metab* 76:309–317, Feb 1993.

Bianda T, Glatz Y, Bouillon R, Froesch ER, Schmid C. (Division of Endocrinology and Metabolism, University Hospital, Zurich, Switzerland.) "Effects of short-term insulin-like growth factor-1 (IGF-1) or growth hormone (GH) treatment on bone metabolism and on production of 1,25-dihydroxycholecalciferol in GH-deficient adults." *J Clin Endocrinol Metab* 83(1):81–87, Jan 1998.

Binnerts A, Swart GR, Wilson JH, Hoogerbrugge N, Pols HA, Birkenhager JC, Lamberts SW. (Department of Internal Medicine, University Hospital Dijkzigt, Rotterdam, The Netherlands.) "The effect of growth hormone administration in growth hormone deficient adults on bone protein, carbohydrate and lipid homeostasis, as well as on body composition." *Clin Endocrinol (Oxf)* 37:79–87, Jul 1992.

Birkenhager-Gillesse EG, Derksen J, Lagaay AM. (Department of Internal Medicine, Leiden University Hospital, The Netherlands.) "DHEAS in the oldest old, aged 85 and over." *Ann NY Acad Sci* 719:543–552, May 1994.

Bjarnason R, Wickelgren R, Hermansson M, Hammarqvist F, Carlsson B, Carlsson LM. (Department of Medicine, International Pediatric Growth Research Center, Goteborg, Sweden.ragnar.bjarnason@pediat.gu.se) "Growth hormone treatment prevents the decrease in insulin-like growth factor-1 gene expression in patients undergoing abdominal surgery." *J Clin Endocrinol Metab* 83(5):1566–1572, May 1998.

Bodnar AG, Ouellette M, Frolkis M, Holt SE, Chiu CP, Morin GB, Harley CB, Shay JW, Lichtsteiner S, Wright WE. (Geron Corporation, Menlo Park, CA 94025, USA.) "Extension of life-span by introduction of telomerase into normal human cells." *Science* 279(5349):349–352, Jan 1998.

Bouillon R. (Catholic University of Leuven, Laboratory of Experimental Medicine and Endocrinology, Belgium.) "Growth hormone and bone." *Horm Res* 36, Suppl 1:49–55, 1991.

Braga M, Costantini E, Di Francesco A, Gianotti L, Baccari P, Di Carlo V. (Department of Surgery, Scientific Institute Hospital San Raffaele, Milan, Italy.) "Impact of thymopentin on the incidence and severity of postoperative infection: a randomized controlled trial." *Br J Surgery* 81(2):205–208, Feb 1994.

Brien TP, Kallakury BV, Lowry CV, Ambros RA, Muraca PJ, Malfetano JH, Ross JS. (Department of Pathology & Laboratory Medicine, Albany Medical College, New York 12208, USA.) "Telomerase activity in benign endometrium and endometrial carcinoma." *Cancer Res* 57(13):2760–2764, Jul 1997.

Brixen K, Kassem M, Nielsen HK, Loft AG, Flyvbjerg A, Mosekilde L. (Department of Endocrinology and Metabolism, Aarhus University Hospital, Denmark.) "Short-term treatment with growth hormone stimulates osteoblastic and osteoclastic activity in osteopenic post-menopausal women: a dose response study." *J Bone Miner Res* 10(12):1865–1874, Dec 1995.

Brody J. "Restoring Ebbing Hormones May Slow Aging." *The New York Times* B5–6, 18 July 1995.

Bryan TM, Reddel RR. (Children's Medical Research Institute, Wentworthville, N.S.W, Australia.) "Telomere dynamics and telomerase activity in in vitro immortalised human cells." *Eur J Cancer* 33(5):767–773, Apr 1997.

Burgstiner CB. "Cure for hepatitis? 'Physician, heal thyself,' and he did." *J Med Assoc Ga* 80(1):21–22, Jan 1991.

Byrne TA, Morrissey TB, Nattakom TV, Ziegler TR, Wilmore DW. (Department of Surgery, Brigham & Women's Hospital, Harvard Medical School, Boston, MA 02115, USA.) "Growth hormone, glutamine, and a modified diet enhance nutrient absorption in patients with severe short bowel syndrome." *J Parenter Enteral Nutr* 19(4):296–302, Jul 1995.

Camanni F, Ghigo E, Arvat E. (Department of Internal Medicine, University of Turin, Italy.) "Growth hormone-releasing peptides." *Euro J Endocrinol* 136(5):445–460, May 1997.

Camanni F, Ghigo E, Arvat E. (Department of Internal Medicine, University of Turin, Italy.) "Growth hormone-releasing peptides and their analogs." *Front Neuroendocrinol* 19(1):47–72, Jan 1998.

Capaldo B, Lembo G, Rendina V, Vigorito C, Guida R, Cuocolo A, Fazio S, Sacca L. (Department of Internal Medicine, IRCCS, NEUROMED, Pozzilli Isernia, Italy.) "Sympathetic deactivation by growth hormone treatment in patients with dilated cardiomyopathy." *Eur Heart J* 19(4):623–627, Apr 1998.

Carter HB, Pearson JD, Metter EJ, Chan DW, Andres R, Fozard JL, Rosner W, Walsh PC. (Department of Urology, James Buchanan Brady Urological Institute, Johns Hopkins Hospital, Johns Hopkins University School of Medicine, Baltimore, MD 21287-2101, USA.) "Longitudinal evaluation of serum androgen levels in men with and without prostate cancer." *Prostate* 27(1):25–31, Jul 1995.

Carter HB, Pearson JD, Waclawiw Z, Metter EJ, Chan DW, Guess HA, Walsh PC. (Department of Urology, James Buchanan Brady Urological Institute, Johns Hopkins Hospital, Johns Hopkins

University School of Medicine, Baltimore, Maryland, USA.) "Prostate-specific antigen variability in men without prostate cancer: effect of sampling interval on prostate-specific antigen velocity." *Urology* 45(4):591–596, Apr 1995.

Cheek DB, Hill DE. "Effect of Growth Hormone on Cell and Somatic Growth." *Handbook of Physiology: A Critical Comprehensive Presentation of Physiological Knowledge and Concepts—Section 7:2 Endocrinology—Part 1: Female Reproductive System.* Greep RO, Astwood EB, eds. Washington: American Physiological Society, 4(7):159–185, 1973.

Christ ER, Carroll PV, Russell-Jones DL, Sonksen PH. (Division of Medicine (UMDS), St. Thomas' Hospital, London.) "The consequences of growth hormone deficiency in adulthood, and the effects of growth hormone replacement." *Schweiz Med Wochenschr* 127(35): 1440–1449, 30 Aug 1997.

Christensen H, Flyvbjerg A, Orskov H, Laurberg S. (Department of Connective Tissue Biology, University of Aarhus, Denmark.) "Effect of growth hormone on the inflammatory activity of experimental colitis in rats." *Scand J Gastronenterol* 28(6):503–511, Jun 1993.

Clark LC, Combs GF Jr, Turnbull BW, Slate EH, Chalker DK, Chow J, Davis LS, Glover RA, Graham GF, Gross EG, Krongrad A, Lesher JL Jr, Park HK, Sanders BB Jr, Smith CL, Taylor JR. (Arizona Cancer Center, College of Medicine, University of Arizona, Tucson, USA.) "Effects of selenium supplementation for cancer prevention in patients with carcinoma of the skin, a randomized controlled trial. Nutritional prevention of cancer study group." *J Am Med Assoc* 276(24):1957–1963, Dec 1996.

Cleary MP. (Hormel Institute, University of Minnesota, Austin 55912.) "The antiobesity effect of dehydroepiandrosterone in rats." *Proc Soc Exp Biol Med* 196(1):8–16, Jan 1991.

Conant MA, Calabrese LH, Thompson SE, et al. "Maintenance of CD4+ cells by thymopentin in asymptomatic HIV-infected subjects: results of a double-blind, placebo-controlled study." *AIDS* 6(11):1335–1339, 1992.

Crook TH, Petrie W, Wells C, Massari DC. (Memory Assessment Clinics, Inc., Bethesda, MD 20814.) "Effects of phosphatidylserine in Alzheimer's disease." *Psychopharmacol Bull* 28:61–66, 1992.

Crook TH, Tinklenberg J, Yesavage J, Petrie W, Nunzi MG, Massari DC. (Memory Assessment Clinics, Inc., Bethesda, MD 20814.) "Effects of phosphatidylserine in age-associated memory impairment." *Neurology* 41:644–649, May 1991.

Cuneo RC, Salomon F, Wiles CM, Hesp R, Sonksen PH. (Division of Medicine, United Medical School, Guy's Hospital, London, United Kingdom.) "Growth hormone treatment in growth hormone-deficient adults: I. Effects on muscle mass and strength." *J Appl Physiol* 70:688–694, Feb 1991.

Dan AJ, Graham EA, Beecher CP, eds. *The Menstrual Cycle*. New York: Springer Publishing Co, 1980.

Danese C, Zavattaro E, Calisi L, Marciano F, Perego MA. (Clinica Medica II, Universita degli Studi di Roma La Sapienza, Italy.) "Long-term thymopentin treatment in systemic scleroderma." *Curr Med Res Opin* 13(4):195–201, 1994.

Davison R, Koets P, Snow WG, Gabrielson LG. "Effects of delta 5 pregnenolone in rheumatoid arthritis." *Arch Int Med* 85:365–388, 1950.

de Boer H, Blok GJ, Voerman B, Derriks P, van der Veen E. (Department of Endocrinology, Free University Hospital, Amsterdam, The Netherlands.) "Changes in subcutaneous and visceral fat mass during growth hormone replacement therapy in adult men." *Int J Obes Relat Metab Disord* 20(6):580–587, Jun 1996.

De la Cruz CP, Revilla E, Rodriguez-Gomez JA, Vizuete ML, Cano J, Machado A. (Departamento de Bioquimica, Bromatologia y Toxicologia, Faculad de Farmacia, Universidad de Sevilla, Spain.) "Deprenyl treatment restores serum insulin-like growth factor-1 (IGF-1) levels in aged rats to young rat level." *Eur J Pharmacol* 327(2–3):215–220, May 1997.

De Ritter E. "Nutritional Requirements of the Master Athlete: Preventive and Orthopedic Problems in Sports Medicine." Third Annual U.C. Irvine CME Program on Sports Medicine, Feb 13–14, 1987.

Dollins AB, Zhdanova IV, Wurtman RJ, Lynch HJ, Deng MH. (Department of Brain and Cognitive Sciences, Massachusetts Institute of Technology, Cambridge 02139.) "Effect of inducing nocturnal serum melatonin concentrations in daytime on sleep, mood, body temperature, and performance." *Proc Natl Acad Sci USA* 91:1824–1828, Mar 1994.

Eckert K, Schmitt M, Garbin F, Wahn U, Maurer HR. (Institute of Pharmacy, Free University of Berlin, Germany.) "Thymosin-alpha 1 effects, in vitro, on lymphokine-activated killer cells from patients with primary immunodeficiencies: preliminary results." *Int J Immunopharmacology* 16(12):1019–1025, Dec 1994.

Ehrenstein D. "Immortality gene discovered." *Science* 279:177, Jan 1998.

Ettinger B, Friedman GD, Bush T, Quesenberry CP Jr. (Division of Research, Kaiser Permanente Medical Care Program, Oakland, California, USA.) "Reduced mortality associated with long-term post-menopausal estrogen therapy." *Obstet Gynecol* 87(1):6–12, Jan 1996.

Fiasche R, Fideleff HL, Moisezowicz J, Frieder P, Pagano SM, Holland M. (Endocrinology Unit, T. Alvarez Hospital, Buenos Aires, Argentina.) "Growth hormone neurosecretory dysfunction in major depressive illness." *Psychoneuroendocrinology* 20(7):727–733, 1995.

Flood JF, Morley JE, Roberts E. (Geriatric Research Education and Clinical Center, Veterans Administration Medical Center, St. Louis, MO 63106, USA.) "Memory-enhancing effects in male mice of pregnenolone and steroids metabolically derived from it." *Proc Natl Acad Sci USA* 89(5):1567–1571, Mar 1992.

Flood JF, Morley JE, Roberts E. (Geriatric Research Education and Clinical Center, Veterans Administration Medical Center, St. Louis, MO 63106, USA.) "Pregnenolone sulfate enhances post-training memory processes when injected in very low doses into limbic system structures: the amygdala is by far the most sensitive." *Proc Natl Acad Sci USA* 92(23):10806–10810, Nov 1995.

Flood JF, Smith GE, Roberts E. (Psychobiology Research Laboratory, Veterans Administration Hospital, Sepulveda, CA

91343.) "DHEA and its sulfate enhance memory retention in mice." *Brain Res* 447(2):269–278, May 1988.

Fossel M. (Department of Medicine, Michigan State University College of Human Medicine, East Lansing, USA. Mfossel@aol.com) "Telomerase and the aging cell: implications for human health." *JAMA* 279(21):1732–1735, Jun 1998.

Fraser WD, Biggart EM, O'Reilly DS, Gray HW, McKillop JH, Thomson JA. (Department of Medicine, University Hospital, Basel, Switzerland.) "Are biochemical tests of thyroid function of any value in monitoring patients receiving thyroxine replacement?" *Br Med J* (Clip Res Ed) 293:808–810, Sep 1986.

Freeman H, Pincus G, Bachrach S, et al. "Therapeutic efficacy of delta 5 pregnenolone in rheumatoid arthritis." *J Am Med Assoc* 143:338–344, 1950.

Frustaci A, Perrone GA, Gentiloni N, Russo MA. (Institute of Cardiology, Catholic University, Rome, Italy.) "Reversible dilated cardiomyopathy due to growth hormone deficiency." *Am J Clin Pathol* 97:503–511, Apr 1992.

Fujita K, Terada H, Ling LZ. (Department of Urology, Hamamatsu University School of Medicine.) "Male sexual insufficiency." *Nippon Rinsho* 55(11):2908–2913, Nov 1997.

Gambrell RD, Maier RC, Sanders BI. "Decreased incidence of breast cancer in post-menopausal estrogen-progestogen users." *Obstet Gynecol* 62(4):435–443, Oct 1983.

Ghiron LJ, Thompson JL, Holloway L, Hintz RL, Butterfield GE, Hoffman AR, Marcus R. (Aging Study Unit, VA Medical Center, Palo Alto, California, USA.) "Effects of recombinant insulin-like growth factor-1 and growth hormone on bone turnover in elderly women." *J Bone Miner Res* 10(12):1844–1852, Dec 1995.

Gluckman P, Klempt N, Guan J, Mallard C, Sirimanne E, Dragunow M, Klempt M, Singh K, Williams C, Nikolics K. (Department of Paediatrics, University of Auckland, New Zealand.) "A role for IGF-1 in the rescue of CNS neurons following hypoxic-ischemic injury." *Biochem Biophys Res Commun* 182(2):593–599, Jan 1992.

Govorin NV, Stupina OP. "Use of thymic peptide thymalin in the complex treatment of therapy-resistant schizophrenia." *Zh Nevropatol Psikhiatr Im S S Korsakova* 90(3): 100–103, 1990.

Grinspoon SK, Baum HB, Peterson S, Klibanski A. (Neuroendocrine Unit, Massachusetts General Hospital, Boston 02114, USA.) "Effects of rhIGF-1 administration on bone turnover during short-term fasting." *J Clin Invest* 96(2):900–906, Aug 1995.

Guth L, Zhang Z, Roberts E. (Department of Biology, College of William and Mary, Williamsburg, VA 23187.) "Key role for pregnenolone in combination therapy that promotes recovery after spinal cord injury." *Proc Natl Acad Sci USA* 91(12):308–312, Dec 1994.

Hansen C. *Grape Seed Extract: Procyanidolic Oligomers (PCO).* New York: Healing Wisdom Publications, 1995.

Hargrove JT, Maxson WS, Wentz AC, Burnett LS. (Department of Obstetrics and Gynecology, Vanderbilt University Medical Center, Nashville, Tennessee.) "Menopausal hormone replacement therapy with continuous daily oral micronized estradiol and progesterone." *Obstet Gynecol* 73:606–612, Apr 1989.

Hays E, Beardsley T. "Immunologic effects of human thymic stromal graft and cell lines."

Clin Immunol Immunopath 33:381, Dec 1984.

Hertoghe T. "Growth Hormone Therapy in Aging Adults." 1996 Annual Conference on Antiaging Medicine and Biomedical Technology, Las Vegas, Nevada.

Hirschberg R. (Division of Nephrology and Hypertension, Harbor-UCLA Medical Center, Torrance 90509.) "Effects of growth hormone and IGF-1 on glomerular ultra filtration in growth hormone-deficient rats." *Regul Pept* 48(1–2):241–250, Oct 1993.

Hwu CM, Kwok CF, Lai TY, Shih KC, Lee TS, Hsiao LC, Lee SH, Fang VS, Ho LT. (Section of Endocrinology and Metabolism, Veterans General Hospital, Taipei, Taiwan, Republic of China.) "Growth hormone (GH) replacement reduces total body fat and normalizes insulin sensitivity in GH-deficient adults: a report of one-year clinical experience." *J Clin Endocrinol Metab* 82(10):3285–3292, Oct 1997.

Iannoli P, Miller JH, Ryan CK, Gu LH, Ziegler TR, Sax HC. (Department of Surgery and Pathology, University of Rochester Medical Center, N.Y. 14642-8410, USA.) "Epidermal growth factor and human growth hormone accelerate adaptation after massive enterectomy in an additive, nutrient-dependent, and site-specific fashion." *Surgery* 122(4):721–728, Oct 1997.

Irwin M, Mascovich A, Gillin JC, Willoughby R, Pike J, Smith TL. "Partial sleep deprivation reduces natural killer cell activity in humans." *Psychosom Med* 56(6):493–498, Nov 1994.

Isidori A, Lo Monaco A, Cappa M. "A study of growth hormone release in man after oral administration of amino acids." *Curr Med Res Opin* 7:475–481, 1981.

Jardieu P, Clark R, Mortensen D, Dorshkind K. (Department of Immunology, Genentech, Inc., South San Francisco, CA 94080.) "In vivo administration of insulin-like growth-factor-1 stimulates primary B lymphopoiesis and enhances lymphocyte recovery after bone marrow transplantation." *J Immunol* 152(9):4320–4327, May 1994.

Johansson AG, Burman P, Westermark K, Ljunghall S. (Department of Internal Medicine, University Hospital, Uppsala, Sweden.) "The bone mineral density in acquired growth hormone deficiency correlates with circulating levels of insulin-like growth factor-1." *J Intern Med* 232:447–452, Nov 1992.

Johnson OL, Cleland JL, Lee HJ, Charnis M, Duenas E, Jaworowicz W, Shepard D, Shahzamani A, Jones AJ, Putney SD. (Alkermes, Inc. Cambridge Massachusetts 02139, USA.) "A month-long effect from a single injection of microencapsulated human growth hormone." *Nat Med* 2(7):795–799, Jul 1996.

Johnson OL, Jaworowicz W, Cleland JL, Bailey L, Charnis M, Duenas E, Wu C, Shepard D, Magil S, Last T, Jones AJ, Putney SD. (Alkermes, Inc. Cambridge Massachusetts 02139, USA.) "The stabilization and encapsulation of human growth hormone into biodegradable microspheres." *Pharm Res* 14(6):730–735, Jun 1997.

Jorgensen JO, Pedersen SA, Thuesen L, Jorgensen J, Ingemann-Hansen T, Skakkebaek NE, Christiansen JS. (Second University Clinic of Internal Medicine, Aarhus Kommunehospital, Denmark.)

"Beneficial effects of growth hormone treatment in GH-deficient adults." *Lancet* 1:1221–1225, Jun 1989.

Jospe N, Powell KR. (Department of Pediatrics, University of Rochester, NY 14642.) "Growth hormone deficiency in an 8-year-old girl with human immunodeficiency virus infection." *Pediatrics* 86(2):309–312, Aug 1990.

Kaiser F, Morley JE. (Department of Medicine, St. Louis University School of Medicine, MO 63104.) "Gonadotropins, testosterone and the aging male." *Neuro Aging* 15:559–563, Jul 1994.

Kalimi M, Regelson W, eds. *The Biologic Role of Dehydroepiandrosterone*. New York: Walter de Gruyter, 1990.

Kamikawa T, Kobayashi A, Yamashita T, Hayashi H, Yamazaki N. "Effects of coenzyme Q-10 on exercise tolerance in chronic stable angina pectoris." *Am J Cardiol* 56(4):247–251, Aug 1985.

Kasai K, Kobayashi M, Shimoda S. "Stimulatory effects of oral glycine on human growth hormone secretion." *Metab* 27(2):201–208, Feb 1978.

Kaufman FR, Gomperts ED. (Division of Endocrinology and Metabolism, Childrens Hospital of Los Angeles, University of Southern California School of Medicine 90027.) "Growth failure in boys with hemophilia and HIV infection." *Am J Pediatr Hematol Oncol* 11(3):292–294, 1989.

Kelley KW, Brief S, Westly HJ, Novakofski J, Bechtel PJ, Simon J, Walker EB. "GH3 pituitary adenoma cells can reverse thymic aging in rats." *Proc Natl Acad Sci USA* 83:5663–5667, Aug 1986.

Kemnitz JW, Roecker EB, Weindruch R, Elson DR, Baum ST, Bergman RN. (Department of Medicine, University of Wisconsin, Madison 53715.) "Dietary restriction increases insulin sensitivity and lowers blood glucose in rhesus monkeys." *Am J Physiol* 266(4 Pt 1):E540–547, Apr 1994.

Kinouchi Y, Hiwatashi N, Chida M, Nagashima F, Takagi S, Mackawa H, Toyota T. (Third Department of Internal Medicine, Tohoku University School of Medicine, Sendai, Japan.) "Telomere shortening in the colonic mucosa of patients with ulcerative colitis." *J Gastroenterol* 33(3):343–348, Jun 1998.

Klein I. (Department of Medicine, North Shore University Hospital, Cornell University Medical College, Manhasset, New York 11030.) "Thyroid hormone and the cardiovascular system." *Am J Med* 88(6):631–637, 1990.

Knoll J. (Department of Pharmacology, Semmelweis University of Medicine, Budapest, Hungary.) "History of deprenyl—the first selective inhibitor of monoamine oxidase type B."

Vopr Med Khim 43(6):482–493, Nov 1997.

Knoll J. (Department of Pharmacology, Semmelweis University of Medicine, Budapest, Hungary.) "The pharmacological basis of the beneficial effects of deprenyl in Parkinson's and Alzheimer's diseases." *J Neural Transm Suppl* 40:69–91, 1993.

Knoll J. (Department of Pharmacology, Semmelweis University of Medicine, Budapest, Hungary.) "The striatal dopamine dependency of lifespan in male rats. Longevity study with (-) deprenyl." *Mech Ageing Dev* Dec 46(1–3):237–262, Dec 1988.

Kyo S, Takakura M, Kohama T, Inoue M. (Department of Obstetrics and Gynecology, School of Medicine, Kanazawa University, Ishikawa, Japan. satoruky@med.kanazawa-u.ac.jp) “Telomerase activity in human endometrium.” *Cancer Res* 57(4):610–614, Feb 1997.

Lamartiniere CA, Moore J, Holland M, Barnes S. (Department of Pharmacology and Toxicology, University of Alabama at Birmingham 35294-0019.) “Neonatal genistein chemo prevents mammary cancer.” *Proc Soc Exp Biol Med* 208(1):120–123, Jan 1995.

Laue L, Pizzo PA, Butler K, Cutler GB Jr. (Department of Pediatrics, Georgetown University, Washington, D.C. 20007.) “Growth and neuroendocrine dysfunction in children with acquired immunodeficiency syndrome.” *J Pediatr* 117(4):541–545, Oct 1990.

Laurie MB. *Resistance to Tuberculosis: Experimental Studies in Native and Acquired Defensive Mechanisms.* Cambridge, Mass, Harvard University Press, 1964.

Laursen T, Jorgensen JO, Christiansen JS. (Medical Department M (Diabetes and Endocrinology), Aarhus Kommunehospital, Denmark.) “Metabolic effects of growth hormone administered subcutaneously once or twice daily to growth hormone deficient adults.” *Clin Endocrinol (Oxf)* 41(3):337–343, Sep 1994.

Le Bars PL, Katz MM, Berman N, Itil TM, Freedman AM, Schatzberg AF. (New York Institute for Medical Research, Tarrytown 10591, USA. NYI@HZI.com) “A placebo-controlled, double-blind, randomized trial of an extract of Ginkgo biloba for dementia. North American EGb Study Group.” *JAMA* Oct. 22;278(16):1327–1332, Oct 1997.

Leal-Cerro A, Garcia E, Astorga R, Casanueva FF, Dieguez C. (Department of Endocrinology, Hospital Virgen del Rocio, Sevilla, Spain.) "Growth hormone (GH) responses to the combined administration of GH-releasing hormone plus GH-releasing peptide 6 in adults with GH deficiency." *Eur J Endocrinol* 132(6):712–715, Jun 1995.

Lee JR. "Is natural progesterone the missing link in osteoporosis prevention and treatment?" *Med Hypotheses* 35(4):316–318 , Aug 1991.

Lee JR. *Natural Progesterone: The Multiple Roles of a Remarkable Hormone.* Sebastopol, Calif.: BLL Publishing, 1993.

Lee John R MD.: *What Your Doctor May Not Tell You About Menopause.* New York: Warner Books, 1996.

Lee William H. *Coenzyme Q-10: Is it Our New Fountain of Youth?* New Canaan, Conn.: Keats Publishing, 1987.

Lesourd B. (Laboratoire d'Immunologie du vieillissement, Faculte de Medecine Pitie-Salpetriere, Paris, France.) "Nutrition and immunity in the elderly: modification of immune responses with nutritional treatment." *Am J Clin Nutr* 66(2):478S–484S, Aug 1997.

Levy JB, Husmann DA. (Department of Urology, Mayo Clinic, Rochester, Minnesota 55905, USA.) "Micropenis secondary to growth hormone deficiency: Does treatment with growth hormone alone result in adequate penile growth?" *J Urol* 156(1):214–216, Jul 1996.

Lin YW, Kubota M, Akiyama Y, Sawada M, Furusho. (Department of Pediatrics, Faculty of Medicine, Kyoto University, Japan.) "Measurement of mutation frequency at the HPRT locus in peripheral lymphocytes. Is this a good method to evaluate a cancer risk in pediatric patients?" *Adv Exp Med Biol* 431:681–686, 1998.

Lissoni P, Barni S, Meregalli S, Fossati V, Cazzaniga M, Esposti D, Tancini G. (Divisione di Radioterapia Oncologica, San Gerardo Hospital, Monza, Milan, Italy.) "Modulation of cancer endocrine therapy by melatonin: a phase II study of Tamoxifen plus melatonin in metastatic breast cancer patients progressing under Tamoxifen alone." *Br J Cancer* 71:854–856, Apr 1995.

Lissoni P, Barni S, Tancini G, Ardizzoia A, Rovelli F, Cazzaniga M, Brivio F, Piperno A, Aldeghi R, Fossati D, et al. (Divisione di Radioterapia Oncologica, San Gerardo Hospital, Milan, Italy.) "Immunotherapy with subcutaneous low-dose Interleukin-2 and the pineal indole melatonin as a new effective therapy in advanced cancers of the digestive tract." *Br J Cancer* 67(6):1404–1407, Jun 1993.

Lolic MM, Fiskum G, Rosenthal RE. (Department of Emergency Medicine, Ronald Reagan Institute of Emergency Medicine, Washington, DC, USA.) "Neuroprotective effects of acetyl-L-carnitine after stroke in rats." *Ann Emerg Med* Jun 29(6):758–765, Jun 1997.

Lombardi G, Colao A, Cuocolo A, Longobardi S, Di Somma C, Orio F, Merola B, Nicolai E, Salvatore M. (Department of Endocrinology and Clinical and Molecular Oncology, Federico II University, Naples, Italy.) "Cardiological aspects of growth hormone and insulin-like growth factor-1." *J Pediatr Endocrinol Metab* 10(6):553–560, Nov 1997.

Marin P. (Department of Heart and Lung Diseases, Sahlgrenska University Hospital, Goteborg, Sweden.) "Testosterone and regional fat distribution." *Obesity Res* 3 Suppl 4:609S–612S, Nov 1995.

Marin P, Holmang S, Jonsson L, Sjostrom L, Kvist H, Holm G, Lindstedt G, Bjorntorp P. (Department of Medicine I, Sahlgren's Hospital, University of Goteborg, Sweden.) "The effects of testosterone treatment on body composition and metabolism in middle-aged obese men." *Int J Obes* 16:991–997, Dec 1992.

Markussis V, Beshyah SA, Fisher C, Nicolaides AN, Johnston DG. (Unit of Metabolic Medicine, St. Mary's Hospital Medical School, London, UK.) "Abnormal carotid compliance and distensibility in hypopituitarism." *Lancet* 340:1188–1192, Nov 1992.

Marusich W, De Ritter E, Bauernfeind JC. "Provitamin activity and stability of beta-carotene in margarine." *J Am Oil Chem Soc* 34:217, 1959.

Massey KA, Blakeslee C, Pitkow HS. (Pennsylvania College of Podiatric Medicine, Philadelphia 19107, USA.) "Possible therapeutic effects of growth hormone on wound healing in the diabetic patient." *J Am Podiatr Assoc* 88(1):25–29, Jan 1998.

McGauley GA, Cuneo RC, Salomon F, Sonksen PH. (Department of Medicine, United Medical School, Guy's Hospital, London, UK.) "Psychological well-being before and after growth hormone treatment in adults with growth hormone deficiency." *Horm Res* 33 Suppl 4:52–54, 1990.

Meeker AK, Sommerfeld HJ, Coffey DS. (The James Buchanan Brady Urological Institute, The Johns Hopkins University School of Medicine, Baltimore, Maryland 21287-2101, USA.) "Telomerase is activated in the prostate and seminal vesicles of the castrated rat." *Endocrinology* 137(12):5743–5746, Dec 1996.

Meikle AW, Arver S, Dobs AS, Sanders SW, Rajaram L, Mazer NA. (Department of Medicine, University of Utah, Salt Lake City 84132, USA.) "Pharmacokinetics and metabolism of a permeation-enhanced testosterone transdermal system in hypogonadal men: influence of application site—a clinical research center study." *J Clin Endocrinol Metab* 81(5):1832–1840, May 1996.

Meling TR, Nylen ES. (Department of Medicine, Veterans Affairs Medical Center, Washington, DC, USA.) "Growth hormone deficiency in adults: a review." *Am J Med Sci* 311:153–166, Apr 1996.

Mendelson WB, Slater S, Gold P, Gillin JC. "The effect of growth hormone administration on human sleep: a dose-response study." *Biol Psychiatry* 15:613–616, Aug 1980.

Mesones HL. "Coenzyme Q-10 in psychiatry." *Acta Psiquiatr Psicol Am Lat* 40(3):207–210, Sep 1994.

Metcalfe JA, Parkhill J, Campbell L, Stacey M, Biggs P, Byrd PJ, Taylor MR. (CRC Institute for Cancer Studies, The Medical School, University of Birmingham, Birmingham B15 2TT, UK. TaylorAMRCvaxl.bham.as.uk) "Accelerated telomere shortening in atoxia telangiectasia." *Nat Genetics* 13(3):350, Jul 1996.

Mevorach D, Perrot S, Buchanan NM, Khamashta M, Laoussadi S, Hughes GR, Menkes CJ. (Department of Medicine, Hadassah University Hospital, Mount Scopus, Jerusalem, Israel.) "Appearance of systemic lupus erythematosus after thymectomy: four case reports and review of the literature." *Lupus* 4(1):33–37, Feb 1995.

Miller JF. "Immunological function of the thymus." *Lancet* 2:748, 1961.

Mohr PE, Wang DY, Gregory WM, Richards MA, Fentiman IS. (Imperial Cancer Research Fund, Clinical Oncology Unit, Guy's Hospital, London, UK.) "Serum progesterone and prognosis in operable breast cancer." *Br J Cancer* 73(12):1552–1555, Jun 1996.

Morales AJ, Nolan JJ, Nelson JC, Yen SS. (Department of Reproductive Medicine, University of California School of Medicine, La Jolla 92093-0802.) "Effects of replacement dose of dehydroepiandrosterone in men and women of advancing age." *J Clin Endocrin Metab* 78(6):1360–1367, Jun 1994.

Mowrey DB. *Herbal Tonic Therapies.* New Canaan, Conn: Keats Publishing, 1993.

Mulligan K, Grunfeld C, Hellerstein MK, Neese RA, Schambelan N. (Division of Endocrinology, San Francisco General Hospital, California 94110.) "Anabolic effects of recombinant human growth hormone in patients with wasting associated with human immunodeficiency virus infection." *J Clin Endocrin Metab* 77(4):956–962, Oct 1993.

Murray F. *Ginkgo Biloba: the Amazing 200 Million-Year-Old Healer.* New Canaan, Conn.: Keats Publishing, 1993.

Nass R, Strasburger CJ. (Medical Clinic, Innenstadt University Hospital, Ludwig-Maximilians-Universitat, Munich, Germany.) "Effects of growth hormone treatment on serum lipids and lipoproteins in adults with growth hormone deficiency." *Eur J Endocrinol* 130 Suppl 2:34, 1994.

Nass R, Huber RM, Klauss V, Muller OA, Schopohl J, Strasburger CJ. (Medical Clinic, Innenstadt University Hospital, Ludwig-Maximilians-Universitat, Munich, Germany.) "Effect of growth hormone replacement therapy on physical work capacity and cardiac and pulmonary function in patients with growth hormone deficiency acquired in adulthood." *J Clin Endocrinol Metab* 80:552–557, Feb 1995.

Norrback KF, Enblad G, Erlanson M, Sundstrom C, Roos G. (Departments of Pathology and Oncology, Umea University, Umea, Sweden; and the Department of Oncology and Pathology, Uppsala University, Uppsala, Sweden.) "Telomerase Activity in Hodgkin's Disease." *Blood* 92(2):567–573, Jul 1998.

Novitzky D, Cooper DK, Chaffin JS, Greer AE, De Bault LE, Zuhdi N. (Oklahoma Transplantation Institute, Baptist Medical Center, Oklahoma City 73112.) "Improved cardiac allograft function following triiodothyronine therapy to both donor and recipient." *Transplantation* 49(2):311–316, Feb 1990.

Nyholm HC, Christensen IJ, Nielsen AL. (Gynaekologisk-obstetrisk afdeling, H:S Hvidovre Hospital.) "The prognostic significance of progesterone receptor level in endometrial cancer." *Ugeskr Laeger* 159(5):601–604, Jan 1997.

O'Halloran DJ, Tsatsoulis A, Whitehouse RW, Holmes SJ, Adams JE, Shalet SM. (Department of Diagnostic Radiology, University of Manchester, United Kingdom.) "Increased bone density after recombinant human growth hormone (GH) therapy in adults with isolated GH deficiency." *J Clin Endocrinol Metab* 76:1344–1348, May 1993.

Osaba D, Miller JR. "The lymphoid tissues and immune responses of neonatally thymectomized mice bearing thymus tissue in millipore diffusion chambers." *Jour Exp Med* 119:177, 1964.

O'Shea M, Miller SB, Finkel K, Hammerman MR. (Washington University School of Medicine, St. Louis, Missouri.) "Roles of growth hormone and growth factors in the pathogenesis and treatment of kidney disease." *Curr Opin Nephrol Hypertens* 2(1):67–72, Jan 1993.

Ovesen P, Jorgensen JO, Ingerslev J, Ho KK, Orskov H, Christiansen JS. (Aarhus Kommunehospital, Aarhus, Denmark.) "Growth hormone treatment of subfertile males." *Fertil Steril* 66(2):292–298, Aug 1996.

Paolisso G, Gambardella A, Giugliano D, Galzerano D, Amato L, Volpe C, Balbi V, Varricchio M, D'Onofrio F. (Department of Geriatric Medicine and Metabolic Diseases, II, University of Naples, Italy.) "Chronic intake of pharmacological doses of vitamin E might be useful in the therapy of elderly patients with coronary heart disease." *Am J Clin Nutr* 81:848–852, Apr 1995.

Papadakis MA, Grady D, Black D, Tierney MJ, Gooding GA, Schambelan M, Grunfeld C. (University of California, San Francisco, California, USA.) "Growth hormone replacement in healthy older men improves body composition but not functional ability." *Ann Int Med* 124(8):708–716, Apr 1996.

Parkes TL, Elia AJ, Dickinson D, Hilliker AJ, Phillips JP, Boulianne GL. (Department of Molecular Biology and Genetics, University of Guelph, Ontario, Canada.) "Extension of Drosophila lifespan by overexpression of human SOD1 in motorneurons." *Nat Genet* 19(2):171–174, Jun 1998.

PEPI Trial. (The Writing Group for the PEPI Trial.) "Effects of hormone replacement therapy on endometrial histology in post-menopausal women." *J Am Med Assoc* 275(5):370–375, Feb 1996.

PEPI Trial. (The Writing Group for the PEPI Trial.) "Effects of estrogen or estrogen/progestin regimens on heart disease risk factors in post-menopausal women." *J Am Med Assoc* 273:199–208, Feb 1995.

Perrig WJ, Perrig P, Stahelin HB. (Institute of Psychology, University of Berne, Switzerland.) "The relation between antioxidants and memory performance in the old and very old." *J Am Geriatr Soc* 45(6):718–724, Jun 1997.

Phillips GB, Pinkernell BH, Jing TY. (Department of Medicine, Columbia University College of Physicians and Surgeons, St. Luke's-Roosevelt Hospital Center, New York, NY, USA.) "The association of hypotestosteronemia with coronary artery disease in men." *Arterioscler Thromb* 14:701–706, Nov 1994.

Pierpaoli W, Bulian D, Dall'Ara A, Marchetti B, Gallo F, Morale MC, Tirolo C, Testa N. (INTERBION Foundation for Basic Biomedical Research, Bellinzoma, Switzerland.) "Circadian melatonin and young-to-old pineal grafting postpone aging and maintain juvenile conditions of reproductive functions in mice and rats." *Exp Gerontol* 32(4–5):587–602, Jul 1997.

Pierpaoli W, Regelson W. (Biancalana-Masera Foundation for the Aged, Convention I.N.R.C.A. and University of Ancona, Neuroimmunomodulation Laboratory, Italy.) "Pineal control of aging: effect of melatonin and pineal grafting on aging mice." *Proc Natl Acad Sci USA* 94:787–791, Jan 1994.

Pierpaoli W, Regelson W. *The Melatonin Miracle.* New York: Simon and Schuster, 1995.

Pincus G, Hoagland H. "Effects of administered pregnenolone on fatiguing psychomotor performance." *J Aviat Med* 15:98–115, 1944.

Pincus G, Hoagland H. "Effects of industrial production of the administration of delta 5 pregnenolone to factory workers." *Psychosomatic Med* 7:342–346, 1945.

Powrie J, Weissberger A, Sonksen P. (Division of Medicine, United Medical School of Guy's Hospital, London, England.) "Growth hormone replacement therapy for growth hormone-deficient adults." *Drugs* 49(5):656–663, May 1995.

Prior JC. (Division of Endocrinology and Metabolism, University of British Columbia, Vancouver, Canada.) "Progesterone as a bone-trophic hormone." *Endocrine Revs* 11:386–398, May 1990.

Pritchett JW. (Department of Orthopaedic Surgery, University of Washington, Seattle.)

"L-dopa in the treatment of nonunited fractures." *Clin Orthop* 255:293–300, Jun 1990.

Puhl JL, Brown CH, eds. *The Menstrual Cycle and Physical Activity.* Champaign, Ill.: Human Kinetics Publishers, Inc., 1986.

Rea MA, Phillips MA, Degraffenried LA, eQin Q, Rice RH. (Department of Environmental Toxicology, University of California, Davis 95616-8588, USA.) "Modulation of human epidermal cell response to 2,3,7,8-tetrachlorodibenzo-p-dioxin by epidermal growth factor." *Carcinogenesis* 19(3):479–483, Mar 1998.

Regelson W, Coleman C. *The Superhormone Promise.* New York: Simon and Schuster, 1996.

Reiter RJ, Tan DX, Poeggeler B, Menendez-Pelaez A, Chen LD, Saarela S. (Department of Cellular and Structural Biology, University of Texas Health Science Center, San Antonio 78284-7762.) "Melatonin as a free radical scavenger: implications for aging and age-related diseases." *Ann NY Acad Sci* 719:1–12, May 1994.

Roberts E. (Department of Neurobiochemistry, Beckman Research Institute of the City of Hope, Duarte, CA 91010.) "Pregnenolone-From Selye to Alzheimer and a model of the pregnenolone sulfate binding site on the GABAA receptor." *Biochem Pharmacol* 49(1):1–16, Jan 1995.

Roberts G. "Dehydroepiandrosterone (DHEA) and its sulfate (DHEAS) as neural facilitators: Effects on brain tissue in culture and on memory in young and old mice. Acyclic GMP hypothesis of action of DHEA and DHEAS in nervous system and other tissues." *The Biologic Role of Dehydroepiandrosterone (DHEA).* Kalimi M, Regelson W, eds. New York: Walter de Gruyter, 1990.

Rosen T, Bengtsson BA. (Department of Internal Medicine II, Sahlgrenska Hospital, Goteborg, Sweden.) "Premature mortality due to cardiovascular disease in hypopituitarism."

Lancet 336:285–288, Aug 1990.

Rosen T, Johannsson G, Johansson JO, Bengtsson BA. (Research Centre for Endocrinology and Metabolism, RCEM, Sahlgrenska University Hospital, Goteborg, Sweden.) "Consequences of growth hormone deficiency in adults and the benefits and risks of recombinant human growth hormone treatment." *Horm Res* 43:93–99, 1995.

Roy JA, Sawka CA, Pritchard KI. (Division of Medical Oncology/ Haematology, Toronto-Sunnybrook Regional Cancer Centre, Ontario, Canada.) "Hormone replacement therapy in women with breast cancer. Do the risks outweigh the benefits?" *J Clin Oncol* 14(3):997–1006, Mar 1996.

Rudling M, Norstedt G, Olivecrona H, Reihner E, Gustafsson JA, Angelin B. (Department of Medicine, Karolinska Institutet, Huddinge University Hospital, Sweden.) "Importance of growth hormone for the induction of hepatic low density lipoprotein receptors." *Proc Natl Acad Sci USA* 89:6983–6987, Aug 1992.

Rudman D, Feller AG, Nagraj HS, Gergans GA, Lalitha PY, Goldberg AF, Schlenker RA, Cohn L, Rudman IW, Mattson DE. (Department of Medicine, Medical College of Wisconsin, Milwaukee.) "Effects of human growth hormone in men over 60 years old." *N Eng J Med* 323:1–6, Jul 1990.

Ruehl WW, Entriken TL, Muggenburg BA, Bruyette DS, Griffith WC, Hahn FF. (Deprenyl Animal Health, Overland Park, KS 66210, USA.) "Treatment with L-deprenyl prolongs life in elderly dogs." *Life Sci* 61(11):1037–1044, 1997.

Russell RM. (Jean Mayer US Dept of Agriculture Human Nutrition Research Center on Aging at Tufts University, Boston, MA 02115, USA.) "New views on RDAs for adults." *J Am Diet Assoc* 97(5):515–518, May 1997.

Russell-Jones DL, Weissberger AJ, Bowes SB, Kelly JM, Thomason M, Umpleby AM, Jones RH, Sonksen PH. (Division of Endocrinology and Medicine, United Medical School, Guy's Hospital, London, UK.) "Protein metabolism in growth hormone deficiency, and effects of growth hormone replacement therapy." *Acta Endocrinol* 128 Suppl 2:44–47, Jun 1993.

Russell-Jones DL, Weissberger AJ, Bowes SB, Kelly JM, Thomason M, Umpleby AM, Jones RH, Sonksen PH. (Division of Endocrinology and Medicine, United Medical School, Guy's Hospital, London, UK.) "The effect of growth hormone replacement on serum lipid, lipoproteins, apolipoproteins and cholesterol precursors in adult growth hormone deficiency patients." *Clin Endocrinol* 41:345–350, Apr 1994.

Russell-Jones DL, Weissberger AJ, Bowes SB, Kelly JM, Thomason M, Umpleby AM, Jones RH, Sonksen PH. (Division of Endocrinology and Medicine, United Medical School, Guy's Hospital, London, UK.) "The effects of growth hormone on protein metabolism in adult growth hormone deficient patients." *Clin Endocrinol (Oxf)* 38(4):427–431, Apr 1993.

Saito T, Schneider A, Martel N, Mizumoto H, Bulgay-Moerschel M, Kudo R, Nakazawa H. (Unit of Multistage Carcinogenesis, International Agency for Research on Cancer, World Health Organization, Lyon, France.) "Proliferation-associated regulation of telomerase activity in human endometrium and its potential implication in early cancer diagnosis." *Biochem Biophys Res Commun* 231(3):610–614, 1997.

Salomon F, Cuneo RC, Hesp R, Sonksen PH. (Division of Medicine, United Medical and Dental Schools of Guy's and St. Thomas', St. Thomas' Hospital, London, United Kingdom.) "The effects of treatment with recombinant HGH on body composition and metabolism in adults with growth hormone deficiency." *N Eng J Med* 321:1797–1703, Dec 1989.

Sandstrom R, Svanberg E, Hyltander A, Haglind E, Ohlsson C, Zachrisson H, Berlund B, Lindholm E, Brevinge H, Lundholm K. (Department of Surgery, Sahlgrenska University Hospital, University of Goteborg, Sweden.) "The effect of recombinant human IGF-1 on protein metabolism in post-operative patients without nutrition compared to effects in experimental animals." *Eur J Clin Invest* 25(10):784–792, Oct 1995.

Sano M, Ernesto C, Thomas RG, Klauber MR, Schafer K, Grundman M, Woodbury P, Growdon J, Cotman CW, Pfeiffer E, Schneider LS, Thal LJ. (Department of Neurology, Columbia University College of Physicians and Surgeons, New York, USA.) "A controlled trial of selegiline, alpha-tocopherol, or both as treatment for Alzheimer's disease." *New Engl J Med* 336(17):1216–1222, Apr 1977.

Schambelan M, Mulligan K, Grunfeld C, Daar ES, LaMarca A, Kotler DP, Wang J, Bozzette SA, Breitmeyer JB. (San Francisco General Hospital, CA 94110, USA.) "Recombinant human growth hormone in patients with HIV-associated wasting. A randomized, placebo-controlled trial. Serostim Study Group." *Ann Intern Med* 125(11):873–882, Dec 1996.

Schmidt R, Fazekas F, Reinhart B, Kapeller P, Fazekas G, Offenbacher H, Eber B, Schumacher M, Freidl W. (Department of Neurology, Karl-Franzens University Graz, Austria.) "Estrogen replacement therapy in older women: a neuropsychological and brain MRI study." *J Am Geriatr Soc* 44(11):1307–1313, Nov 1996.

Schmuck A, Ravel A, Coudray C, Alary J, Franco A, Roussel AM. (GREPO, Universite Joseph Fourier, Domaine de la Merci, La Tronche, France.) "Antioxidant vitamins in hospitalized elderly patients: analysed dietary intakes and biochemical status." *Eur J Clin Nutr* 50(7):473–478, Jul 1996.

Schwartz AG, Pashko LL. (Fels Institute for Cancer Research and Molecular Biology, Temple University School of Medicine, Philadelphia, PA 19140.) "Cancer chemoprevention with the adrenocortical steroid dehydroepiandrosterone and structural analogs." *J Cell Biochem* Suppl 17G:73–79, 1993.

Schwartz J, Freeman R, Frishman W. (Department of Medicine, Albert Einstein College of Medicine, Bronx, New York, USA.) "Clinical pharmacology of estrogens: cardiovascular actions and cardioprotective benefits of replacement therapy in post-menopausal women." *J Clin Pharmacol* 35(1):1–16, 35(3):314–329, Jan, Mar 1995.

Shealy NC. *DHEA: The Youth and Health Hormone.* New Canaan: Keats Publishing, Inc., 1996.

Shen XY, Holt RI, Miell JP, et al. "Cirrhotic liver expresses low levels of the full-length

and truncated growth hormone receptors." *J Clin Endocrinol Metab* 83(7):2532–2538,1998.

Sherwin BB. (Department of Psychology, McGill University, Montreal, Quebec, Canada.) "Affective changes with estrogen and androgen replacement therapy in surgically menopausal women." *J Affect Disord* 14(2):177–187, Mar 1988.

Sherwin BB. (Department of Psychology, McGill University, Montreal, Quebec, Canada.) "Estrogen and/or androgen replacement therapy and cognitive functioning in surgically menopausal women." *Psychoneuroendocrinology* 13(4):345–357, 1988.

Sherwin BB. (Department of Psychology, McGill University, Montreal, Quebec, Canada.) "Sex hormones and psychological functioning in post-menopausal women." *Exp Gerontol* 29:423–430, May 1994.

Shinobe M, Sanaka T, Nihei H, Sugino N. (Department of Medicine, Tokyo Women's Medical College, Japan.) "IGF-1/IGFBP-1 as an index for discrimination between responder and nonresponder to recombinant human growth hormone in malnourished uremic patients on hemodialysis." *Nephron* 77(1):29–36, 1997.

Snyder DK, Underwood LE, Clemmons DR. (Department of Medicine, East Carolina University School of Medicine, Greenville, North Carolina 27858-4354.) "Persistent lipolytic effect of exogenous growth hormone during caloric restriction." *Am J Med* 98(2):129–134, Feb 1995.

Sonntag WE, Forman LJ, Miki N, Trapp JM, Gottschall PE, Meites J. "L-dopa restores amplitude of growth hormone pulses in old male rats to that observed in young male rats." *Neuroendocrinology* 34(3):163–168, Mar 1982.

Sonntag WE, Lenham JE, Ingram RL. (Department of Physiology and Pharmacology, Bowman Gray School of Medicine, Winston-Salem, NC 27157-1083.) "Effects of aging and dietary restriction on tissue protein synthesis: relationship to plasma insulin-like growth Factor-1." *J Gerontol* 47(5):B159–163, Sep 1992.

Spagnoli A, Lucca U, Menasce G, Bandera L, Cizza G, Forloni G, Tettamanti M, Frattura L, Tiraboschi P, Comelli M, et al. (Mario Negri Institute for Pharmacological Research, Milan, Italy.) "Long-term acetyl-L-carnitine treatment in Alzheimer's disease." *Neurology* 41(11):1726–1732, Nov 1991.

Stabler SP, Lindenbaum J, Allen RH. (Department of Medicine, University of Colorado Health Sciences Center, Denver 80220, USA. jonesjoCjove.UCHSC.edu) "Vitamin B12 deficiency in the elderly: current dilemmas." *Am J Clin Nutr* 66(4):741–749, Oct 1997.

Stiller MJ, Shupack JL, Kenny C, Jondreau L, Cohen DE, Soter NA. (Ronald O. Perelman Department of Dermatology, New York University School of Medicine, NY.) "A double-blind, placebo controlled clinical trial to evaluate the safety and efficacy of thymopentin as an adjunctive treatment in atopic dermatitis." *J Am Acad Dermatol* 30(4):597–602, Apr 1994.

Stokkan KA, Reiter RJ, Nonaka KO, Lerchl A, Yu BP, Vaughan MK. (Department of Cellular and Structural Biology, University of Texas Health Science Center, San Antonio 78284.) "Food restriction retards aging of the pineal gland." *Brain Res* 545(102):66–72, Apr 1991.

Sundal E, Bertelletti D. (Cilag spa, Cologno Monzese, Italy.) "Management of viral infections with thymopentin." *Arzneimittel-Forschung* 44(7):866–871, Jul 1994.

Sundal E, Bertelletti D. (Cilag spa, Cologno Monzese, Italy.) "Thymopentin treatment of rheumatoid arthritis." *Arzneimittel-Forschung* 44(10):1145–1149, Oct 1994.

Tang MX, Jacobs D, Stern Y, Marder K, Schofield P, Gurland B, Andrews H, Mayeux R. (Gertrude H. Serglevsky Center, Columbia University, New York, NY 10032, USA.) "Effect of oestrogen during menopause on risk and age at onset of Alzheimer's disease." *Lancet* 348:429–432, Aug 1996.

Thompson JL, Butterfield GE, Gylfadottir UK, Yesavage J, Marcus R, Hintz RL, Pearman A, Hoffman AR. (Geriatric Research Education and Clinical Center and Medical Service, Veterans Affairs Health Care System, Palo Alto, California 94304, USA.) "Effects of human growth hormone, insulin-like growth factor-1, and diet and exercise on body composition of obese post-menopausal women." *J Clin Endocrinol Metab* 83(5):1477–1484, May 1998.

Turturro A, Blank K, Murasko D, Hart R. (Division of Biometry and Risk Assessment, National Center for Toxicological Research, Jefferson, Arkansas 72079.) "Mechanisms of caloric restriction affecting aging and disease." *Ann NY Acad Sci* 719:159–170, May 1994.

van Vollenhoven RF, Morabito LM, Engleman EG, McGuire JL. (Division of Immunology and Rheumatology, Stanford University Medical Center, CA 94305-5111, USA.) "Treatment of systemic lupus erythematosus with dehydroepiandrosterone: 50 patients treated up to 12 months." *J Rheumatol* 25(2):285–289, Feb 1998.

Verhelst J, Abs R, Vandeweghe M, Mockel J, Legros JJ, Copinschi G, Mahler C, Velkeniers B, Vanhaelst L, Van Aelst A, De Rijdt D, Stevenaert A, Beckers A. (Department of Endocrinology, Algemeen Ziekenhuis Middelheim, Antwerpen, Belgium.) "Two years of replacement therapy in adults with growth hormone deficiency." *Clin Endocrinol (Oxf)* 47(4):485–494, Oct 1997.

Wahlin A, Backman L, Hill RD, Winblad B. (Karolinska Institutet.) "Measurement of folic acid and vitamin B12 in the elderly. Low serum levels result in worse memory." *Lakaertidningen* 94(23):2177–2182, Jun 1997.

Walford RL, Harris SB, Gunion MW. (Space Biospheres Ventures, Oracle, AZ 85623.) "The calorically restricted low-fat nutrient-dense diet in Biosphere 2 significantly lowers blood glucose, total leukocyte count, cholesterol, and blood pressure in humans." *Proc Natl Acad Sci USA* 89(23):11533–37, Dec 1992.

Weideger P. *Menstruation and Menopause: The Physiology and Psychology, the Myth and the Reality.* New York: Alfred A. Knopf, 1976.

Weindruch R, Walford RL, Fligiel S, Guthrie D. "The retardation of aging in mice by dietary restriction: longevity, cancer, immunity and lifetime energy intake." *J Nutr* 116(4):641–654, Apr 1986.

Weiss NS. (University of Washington, Seattle 98195, USA. nweiss@a u.washington.edu) "Health consequences of short- and long-term post-menopausal hormone therapy." *Clin Chem* 42(8 Pt 2):1342–1344, Aug 1996.

Whitehead HM, Boreham C, McIlrath EM, Sheridan B, Kennedy L, Atkinson AB, Hadden

DR. (Sir George E. Clark Metabolic Unit, Royal Victoria Hospital, Belfast, UK.) "Growth hormone treatment of adults with growth hormone deficiency: results of a 13-month placebo controlled cross-over study." *Clin Endocrinol (Oxf)* 36:45–52, Jan 1992.

Windisch PA, Papatheofanis FJ, Matuszewski KA. (Clinical Practice Advancement Center, University HealthSystem Consortium, Oak Brook, IL 60521, USA. windisch@msgate.uhc.edu) "Recombinant human growth hormone for AIDS-associated wasting." *Ann Pharmacother* 32(4):437–445, Apr 1998.

Wolkowitz OM, Reus VI, Roberts E, Manfredi F, Chan T, Ormiston S, Johnson R, Canick J, Brizendine L, Weingartner H. (Department of Psychiatry, UCSF 94143-0984, USA.) “Antidepressant and cognition-enhancing effects of DHEA in major depression.” *Ann NY Acad Sci* 774:337–339, Dec 1995.

Wolkowitz OM, Reus VI, Roberts E, Manfredi F, Chan T, Raum WJ, Ormiston S, Johnson R, Canick J, Brizendine L, Weingartner H. (Department of Psychiatry, University of California, San Francisco, School of Medicine 94143-0984, USA.) “Dehydroepiandrosterone (DHEA) treatment of depression.” *Biol Psychiatry* 41(3):311–318, Feb 1997.

Wuster C, Slenczka E, Ziegler R. (Abteilung Innere Medizin I, Endokrinologie and Stoffwechsel, Universitat Heidelberg.) “Increased prevalence of osteoporosis and arteriosclerosis in conventionally substituted anterior pituitary insufficiency: need for additional growth hormone substitution?” *Klin Wochenschr* 69(16):769–773, Oct 1991.

Yamanouchi T, Moromizato H, Kojima S, et al. “Prevention of diabetes by thymic hormone in alloxan-treated rats.” *Eur J Pharmacol* 257(1–2):39–46, 1994.

Yang R, Bunting S, Gillett N, Clark RG, Jin H. (Department of Cardiovascular Research, Genentech, Inc., South San Francisco 94080, USA.) “Effects of growth hormone in rats with postinfarction left ventricular dysfunction.” *Cardiovasc Drugs Ther* 9(1):125–131, Feb 1995.

Yokoyama Y, Takahashi Y, Morishita S, Hashimoto M, Niwa K, Tamaya T. (Department of Obstetrics and Gynecology, Gifu University School of Medicine, Japan.) “Telomerase activity in the human endometrium throughout the menstrual cycle." *Mol Hum Reprod* 4(2):173–177, Feb 1998.

Zhao X, Unterman TG, Donovan SM. (Division of Foods and Nutrition, University of Illinois, Urbana 61801, USA.) "Human growth hormone but not human insulin-like growth factor-1 enhances recovery from neonatal malnutrition in rats." *J Nutr* 125(5):1316–1327, May 1995.

Zhdanova IV, Wurtman RJ, Lynch HJ, Ives JR, Dollins AB, Morabito C, Matheson JK, Schomer DL. (Clinical Research Center, Massachusetts Institute of Technology, Cambridge 02142, USA.) "Sleep-inducing effects of low doses of melatonin ingested in the evening." *Clin Pharmacol Ther* 57:552–558, May 1995.

Zubialde JP, Lawler F, Clemenson N. (Department of Family Medicine, University of Oklahoma Health Sciences Center, Oklahoma City 73104.) "Estimated gains in life expectancy with use of post-menopausal estrogen therapy: a decision analysis." *J Fam Prac* 36:271–289, Mar 1993.